Fitness for Travelers

Also by Suzanne Schlosberg

The Ultimate Workout Log:
An Exercise Diary and Fitness Guide

Fitness for Dummies,
with Liz Neporent

Weight Training for Dummies,
with Liz Neporent

Fitness for Travelers

The Ultimate Workout Guide for the Road

Suzanne Schlosberg

Houghton Mifflin Company

Boston · New York

2002

RA
776
.S3293
2002

Visit our Web site: www.houghtonmifflinbooks.com.

Library of Congress Cataloging-in-Publication
Data is available.

ISBN 0-618-11592-7 (pbk.)

Printed in the United States of America

Book design by Joyce C. Weston

RRD 10 9 8 7 6 5 4 3 2 1

Photographs courtesy of Covey Media

To Grandma Ruth, a road warrior

Contents

Final Thoughts 174

About the Authors

Suzanne Schlosberg

Suzanne Schlosberg is a health, fitness, and humor writer who lives in Los Angeles. A contributing editor to Shape magazine, she is the author of *The Ultimate Workout Log* and the coauthor, with Liz Neporent, of *Fitness for Dummies* and *Weight Training for Dummies*. She is also a journalism instructor at UCLA Extension. Always happy with a barbell in hand, Schlosberg hunts for gyms wherever she travels, from Alaska to Zimbabwe, New Orleans to New Guinea. She is the women's record holder in the Great American Sack Race, a quadrennial event held in Yerington, Nevada, in which competitors run 5 miles while carrying a 50-pound sack of chicken feed. The 22-inch trophy remains her crowning, and only, achievement in the realm of athletic competition. Schlosberg is also a road-bike racer who holds her cycling club's record for most meals eaten at Denny's on a weekend road trip: 5, in 38 hours. Suzanne has cycled across the United States twice, stopping frequently to lift weights and eat at Dairy Queen. She can be reached at schlos1@aol.com.

The American Council on Exercise

The American Council on Exercise (ACE) is a nonprofit organization dedicated to promoting the benefits of physical activity and protecting consumers against unsafe and ineffective fitness products and instructions. As the nation's "workout watchdog," ACE conducts university-based research and testing that targets fitness products and trends. ACE sets standards for fitness professionals and is the world's largest non-profit fitness certifying organization. For more information on ACE and its programs, call (800) 825-3636 or log onto the ACE Web site at www.acefitness.org.

Expert Contributors

Ken Alan, who designed the hotel-room strength workouts in Chapter 12, is a spokesperson for the American Council on Exercise (ACE) and is certified by the American College of Sports Medicine (ACSM) and the Aerobics and Fitness Association of America (AFAA). Formerly director of employee fitness at Cedars-Sinai Medical Center in Los Angeles, Alan now travels extensively, presenting workshops for fitness professionals. He is also a guest faculty member at UCLA Extension and Cal State Fullerton University Extension. A recipient of IDEA's Instructor of the Year award, Alan owns AeroBeat Music & Video. He can be reached at kenalanfitness@aol.com.

Ken Baldwin, M.A., who designed the multi-gym workouts in Chapter 9, is an ACE-certified trainer and president of Premier Fitness Inc., a personal training business based in San Diego. He is the former chairman of the Senior Fitness Committee, a former member of the Massachusetts Governor's Committee on Physical Fitness and Sports, and former chairman of IDEA's National Personal Trainer Committee. Baldwin was the winner of the 1999 IDEA Personal Trainer of the Year award. He can be reached at ken@premierfitness.com or www.premierfitness.com.

Scott Cole, who designed the yoga and tai chi workout in Chapter 14, has entertained audiences in more than thirty countries as a fitness and wellness presenter and motivational speaker, as a National Aerobic Champion, and as a star of Abs of Steel videos. Cole's newest videos — *Tai Chi Training, Millennium Stretch, Yin/Yang Workout,* and *The Best Abs on Earth* — reflect his slogan of "Lifting spirits and buttocks to new heights." Based in Palm Springs, California, Cole is dedicated to bringing the martial and healing arts into schools, senior centers, and health clubs worldwide. For more on Cole, visit www.scottcole.com.

Christine "CC" Cunningham, M.S., who designed the cardio workouts in Chapter 6, serves on the ACE Faculty Board of Advisors and is a Certified Athletic Trainer and Certified Strength and Conditioning Coach. The owner of performENHANCE, a sports and adventure athlete training company, Cunningham specializes in applying advanced conditioning methods to exercise programs. She competes in both mountain biking and cyclocross events and is an avid trail runner, hiker, cross-country skier, and rock climber. Cunningham is working on her Ph.D. in exercise neuroscience at the University of Illinois at Chicago. She can be reached at performenhance@aol.com.

Troy DeMond, M.A., who designed the tubing workouts in Chapter 11, is an ACE-certified trainer and the owner of Fitness On The Move Lifestyle Center in Fort Myers, Florida. He has created and starred in six top-rated exercise videos, including *Pump I.T. with Troy DeMond, M.A.* and *Troy DeMond's TNT Workout.* He is the author of two fitness books and has traveled to more than fifteen countries, lecturing to fitness enthusiasts and professionals. He is also the national spokesperson for Spri Products. DeMond can be reached at fitonmove@myexcel.com.

Liz Neporent, M.A., who designed the dumbbell workouts in Chapter 10, is a corporate fitness consultant who designs and manages fitness centers worldwide for Plus One Fitness in New York City. She is certified by ACE, ACSM, the National Strength and Conditioning Association, and the National Academy of Sports Medicine. Neporent also serves on the ACE board of directors and was recently named Club Industry Magazine's Woman Entrepreneur of the Year. She is the co-author and author of several books, including *Fitness for Dummies, Fitness Walking for Dummies,* and *Weight Training for Dummies.* Neporent can be reached at lizzyfit@aol.com.

Kerry O'Brien, who designed the swimming workouts in Chapter 7, is the head coach of northern California's Walnut Creek Masters Swim Team, the winningest team in United States Masters history. O'Brien has been selected for the United States Masters Swimming coaching staff at the Olympic Training Center and provides Mentor Coaching around the country for United States Masters Swimming.

Angie Proctor, who designed the aquatic workouts in Chapter 7, is executive director of the Aquatic Exercise Association and president of Personal Body Trainers, Inc., which specializes in advanced land and water applications. Proctor has produced more than 30 aquatic fitness videos and is a leading international presenter on fitness, marketing, and management. She serves as an adviser to Promise Enterprises, Dynamix Music, and the AquaTrend Water Workout Station. Her certifications include ACE, AFAA, the Florida Institute of Back Safety, and the Institute of Aerobic Research. Proctor, who lives in Nokomis, Florida, can be reached at dangie@gte.net.

Tom Seabourne, Ph.D., who designed the stretching workout in Chapter 13, holds certifications from ACE, ACSM, and the United States Professional Tennis Association, and he is a Certified Strength and Conditioning Specialist. He is a two-time all-American in tae kwon do and a two-time national AAU heavyweight tae kwon do champion, North American champion, Pan-American champion, and world silver medalist. A top-ten finisher in the Race Across America, Seabourne holds several ultra-endurance cycling records. His latest book and video, *The Best Abs on Earth*, is written and produced with Scott Cole. Seabourne can be reached at www.onlinetofitness.com.

Ellie Zografakis, R.D., who contributed to Chapter 4, is a registered dietitian and ACE-certified personal trainer. She is also the cofounder of Nutriformance gyms in St. Louis, Missouri, with a staff of personal trainers, registered dietitians, massage therapists, and physical therapists. Zografakis specializes in sports and cardiovascular nutrition, eating disorders, weight loss, and weight maintenance. She lectures nationally on sports nutrition, eating disorders, family nutrition, and basic nutrition to various athletic teams, schools, and corporations. She can be reached at elliez@mail.nutriformance.com.

Acknowledgments

I'm especially grateful to my editor, Susan Canavan, for her enthusiasm and insightful comments, and to my agent, Felicia Eth, for her persistence.

A big thanks to Christine Ekeroth and Ken Germano for involving ACE in this project and to Christine for coordinating many aspects of it. I'm also indebted to research assistants Jennifer Schiffer, Jenna Ferer, and Casie Kesterson, who were relentless in their pursuit of elusive information.

I owe a lot to the fitness professionals who generously contributed their time, creative ideas, and expertise: Ken Alan, Ken Baldwin, Scott Cole, Troy DeMond, CC Cunningham, Kerry O'Brien, Angie Proctor, Tom Seabourne, and Ellie Zografakis. Liz Neporent deserves her own sentence for always coming to my rescue.

The ACE team of reviewers — Richard Cotton, Christine Ekeroth, Dan Green, Shay McKelvey, and, most significantly, CC Cunningham — greatly improved the manuscript. For their work on the photo shoot, my gratitude goes to Karen McGuire, Dennis Dal Covey, and Jim Freeman, as well as to Tony Ordas and Monica Schrader. The models — Fred Elias, Dave Murphy, Carolyn Ryba, and DeeDee Kovacevich — were great sports. Thanks, also, to the Fitness Warehouse in San Diego for letting us use the store for our shoot.

I appreciate the input of the dozens of ACE trainers who filled out our surveys, especially Michael Gavino, Brian Hasenbauer, Mary Hetherington, Kevin Lee, Joanne Maybeck, Jim Wilson, and Adita Yrizarry. I also got some help from my friends, including Nancy Kruh, who offered astute comments, and Allan St. Pierre, who helped with product testing. Finally, thanks to all the fit travelers I interviewed for sharing your tales, ideas, and tips.

— S.S.

Fitness for Travelers

Introduction

You can trace the idea for this book back to my 1999 workout at what may be the world's most inadequate gym, located in the basement of an overpriced hotel in Marrakesh. In the ten days I'd been touring Morocco, I hadn't managed a decent session of exercise. When I wasn't slouched on a train or a bus, I was trudging in 97-degree heat to a famous tomb, or lying under a hotel-room fan and whining about the weather. The only time I'd gotten my heart rate near the aerobic zone was during an argument with a lunatic rug salesman.

The lack of exercise was making me feel grumpy and rundown, so when I happened by a hotel that advertised its FITNESS CENTER on a large sign, I was thrilled. Air conditioning! A stairclimber! A rack full of dumbbells! Alas, what I found — *after* handing over my credit card — was a small stuffy room with a collection of America's most disgraced infomercial exercise gadgets. There was a plastic, triangular abdominal gizmo that resembled a model of the starship *Enterprise*. There was a ThighMaster. There was a treadmill with a belt that did not move unless you propelled it yourself, a very scary piece of machinery that would have collapsed under the weight of Kate Moss.

My instinct was to blow off the workout. Between the flimsy equipment and my general feeling of lethargy, I had a couple of decent excuses. But then I rallied. I figured, Better to make do with a lousy gym than to spend yet another sluglike day gorging on honey-coated pastries. There was a mat on the floor, so I did crunches and pushups. I used the gym's only set of dumbbells for squats and lunges. I sprinted up and down the basement stairs. I stretched. Afterward, I felt much, much better.

You always do when you work out on the road. You feel rejuvenated and more equipped to tackle the day, whether it involves bargaining at

Moroccan rug shops or attending business meetings in Miami. You sleep more soundly, even on a saggy mattress in a motel room that overlooks the freeway. You have more strength for schlepping your luggage. You gain less weight from your airport eating splurges. You're more relaxed and cheerful — and less prone to a meltdown when the rental-car agent informs you that the last available vehicle just drove off the lot.

But staying fit on the road isn't as easy as spotting a FITNESS CENTER sign. It can take ingenuity, resourcefulness, and an extra dose of motivation — even a new set of skills and a whole new mindset. On all these fronts, *Fitness for Travelers* comes to the rescue. This book is for everyone who ever takes a trip: business travelers and vacationers, fitness novices and veterans, tourists going the four-star route or those venturing around on the cheap. You'll find this book useful if:

- You have trouble sustaining a routine on the road because you're too busy, exhausted, or stressed. The book answers your pressing questions: How can I muster the incentive to exercise when I'd rather crash on my hotel bed and watch HBO? How can I minimize jet lag and maximize sleep? How can I possibly fit in exercise when I'm working twelve hours a day? Can I maintain my fitness on two workouts a week?

- You don't have the skills or confidence to exercise in unfamiliar surroundings. Maybe you're comfortable at your local gym but need help adapting your routine to the machines or dumbbells at your hotel. Or maybe you wonder: Can I get a decent strength workout in a motel room? How can I get my heart rate up if the neighborhood is unsafe for jogging? How can I burn calories in a hotel pool that's barely bigger than a hot tub?

- You don't have access to — or interest in — a hotel gym. What's the best way to find a nearby health club that welcomes visitors? How much can you expect to pay for a workout? Which Web sites can help you find a local running route, hiking trail, or Olympic-size pool? What are the best gadgets to pack so you can exercise away from a gym?

For help in answering these questions, I turned to the world's largest organization of fitness professionals, the American Council on Exercise, which has certified more than 100,000 trainers in 77 countries. The workouts in this book were designed by some of ACE's most accomplished, creative, and well-traveled trainers.

But *Fitness for Travelers* gives you more than guidance from the experts. You'll also find useful tips and instructive tales from some of the country's busiest travelers, including touring musicians, commercial pilots, newspaper correspondents, business executives, and political campaign consultants. I spoke to Lynyrd Skynyrd drummer Michael Cartellone, who performs an elaborate strength routine in his hotel room every morning. "I've never let traveling get in the way of my workouts," says Cartellone, who's been known to do pushups on the floor of a moving tour bus. "I'm so focused that I probably get a better workout on the road than I do at home."

Mike Feldman, the traveling chief of staff for Al Gore's 2000 presidential campaign, told me he'd often drag himself out of bed at 5 A.M. to jog. "There was never a time when I finished a run that I wasn't happy I did it," said Feldman, who traveled to four, five, even seven cities a day. "It changes your outlook. It makes you feel healthier and clears your head. I spent all my time in hotels, minivans, and the same airplane, constantly protected by armed federal agents. Jogging was my only chance to get out of the bubble."

Whether you're traveling for business or for fun, exercise is a great way to escape your own bubble — of business meetings, conventions, or sightseeing tours. And who knows what strange and remarkable experiences may await. At a gym in the Russian Far East, I lifted steel weights shaped like bowling balls and clothing irons. At a club in Kenya, I found gigantic handmade weight plates that were so thin they looked like oversize LPs. While on business in Thailand, controller David Negus found an elaborate gym set up in a downtown park. "There were cable pulleys nailed to the branches and weight bars resting on stakes that had been pounded into the trees," says Negus, who has exercised in more than sixty countries while working for international nonprofit organizations.

Sometimes it's not the machines that are intriguing but the people. Once, before visiting Iceland, I used the Internet to track down Albert Jakobsson, president of that country's only road-cycling club. Albert, a thirty-eight-year-old computer technician, kindly offered to lend me a bike and take me on a ride upon my arrival in Reykjavik. He was eager to chat about road-bike racing, a sport that has aroused the passion of exactly seven of his countrymen — cyclists who train year-round, even in subfreezing temperatures, even in the dark, even in the snow.

The day Albert and I rode, temperatures barely topped 30 degrees, winds blew hard, and it rained nonstop. We cycled all of nine miles on a bike path before coming to an abrupt halt where the pavement ended. I was ready to turn around; my clothes were soaked, my toes were numb, and I'd had more than my fill of the Icelandic cycling scene. As we made our way back, I asked Albert why he bothers to ride a road bike in a country that has no decent roads, no road-bike shops, no daylight half the year, and almost no good weather.

"We are Vikings!" he said.

I'm no Viking. I'm just a person who thrives on the energy I get from exercise and the adventure that's often involved in breaking a sweat on the road. I hope this book infuses both energy and adventure into your own travel workouts.

PART I

Adopting the Road Workout Mindset

Even if you work out regularly at home, exercising on the road may seem like a foreign concept. Who has the time? Who has the energy? Who has the suitcase space for workout gear? Exercise may be one habit that you automatically leave at home, along with your nightly Letterman viewing or evening walk with your pooch.

But your workout program is actually quite portable (much more so than, say, your golden retriever). This section prepares you, in several important ways, to exercise on a trip. Chapter 1 gets you in the workout frame of mind, offering strategies to overcome jet lag, fatigue, waning motivation, and other travel workout obstacles. Chapter 2 helps you pack by recommending several small, light gadgets to make your workouts more convenient, more effective, and more comfortable. Chapter 3 — filled with Web site addresses, charts, and tips — helps you locate a place to sweat, whether you're in a big city or a small town, whether you want to swim, jog, or lift weights. Chapter 4 prepares you to navigate the nutritional minefields you may encounter on the road, such as airport restaurants, airline meals, and fast-food joints.

In short, Part I gives you the inspiration, the resources, and the nutritional savvy to stay in shape when you're out of town.

1

Roadblocks: Overcoming the Top Five Travel Workout Obstacles

It's tough enough to squeeze in exercise when you're at home on a consistent schedule. Work, family commitments, and other demands on your time and energy — in other words, life — can distract even the most dedicated exerciser. But travel makes fitness that much tougher to maintain. When you're disoriented from jet lag, stiff from a long flight, stressed out from business meetings, wiped out from sightseeing, baffled by alien exercise equipment or the finer points of a foreign language — or all of the above — staying in shape is an even bigger challenge.

Plus, you have better things to do on your trip than work up a sweat, right? If you're traveling on business, your schedule is probably booked. And if you're traveling for pleasure, well, chances are a hotel treadmill isn't high on your list of must-see tourist attractions.

It's easy to talk yourself out of exercising on the road. But it's also easier than you might think to talk yourself back into it. The key is to anticipate the inevitable roadblocks and be prepared to circumvent them. Know how to schedule your flights, your naps, your exposure to light. Learn how to get work done while you work out. Master the tricks for staying motivated when you'd rather be anywhere but your hotel gym. Expand your repertoire of exercises so you can work out in any location, with any equipment.

Even more important, embark on your trip with a flexible mindset. If you're a regular exerciser at home, you may think that working out on the road is an either-or proposition: either you should complete your usual routine or you shouldn't bother working out at all. But given the unpredictable nature of travel, black-and-white thinking will only leave you frustrated — and set you back when you start exercising again at home. Stay focused on your fitness goals when you travel, but remain realistic, too. Cut yourself slack when your plans go awry.

Although working out on the road may seem like a tall order, some of the world's most frequent flyers manage to run, stretch, and lift weights away from home. Heck, there are even long-haul truckers who sit behind the wheel fourteen hours a day, live on truck-stop food, and still find a way to stay in shape. If they can do it, so can you. This chapter offers solutions for overcoming the five most common travel workout obstacles, along with tips and inspiration from some of the busiest travelers we could find.

Obstacle 1: "I don't have time."

How can you possibly find the time to lift weights or go for a jog when you have meetings to attend, clients to entertain, monuments to marvel at, and desserts to linger over? Here's how.

Exercise first thing in the morning. Wake up earlier than your coworkers or travel companions so you can sweat before the day gets away from you. If that sounds impossible, consider Chris Lehane, who was on the road for nearly two years straight as Al Gore's press secretary for the 2000 presidential campaign. Lehane's workday would start at 6 A.M., when he'd read a half dozen newspapers and prepare for Gore's 6:30 A.M. briefing. Then he'd accompany the vice president from campaign rally to day-care center visit to neighborhood walk to evening fundraiser — each event in a different city. So when did he fit in his daily four-mile jogs? At 5 A.M. "It was really hard to get up, but you just realize you're so much better off for doing it," says Lehane. "It was the one thing I had control over."

> "It was really hard to get up, but you just realize you're so much better off for doing it," says Lehane. "It was the one thing I had control over."

Work while you work out. Read a stack of reports while riding a stationary bike.

Rehearse a sales pitch while you swim. Sex therapist Diana Wiley, host of Hawaii's *Fifty-Plus and Fabulous* radio show, often uses her treadmill time on the road to prepare for conference presentations or upcoming shows. "I'll go over my notes or do my homework for an author interview," says Wiley, 57. "The time goes faster, and I feel like I'm accomplishing two really great things." *Los Angeles Times* White House correspondent Ed Chen, who has traveled with George Bush, Bill Clinton, and George W. Bush, says he does some of his most creative thinking while jogging. "I've worked through writer's block and come up with some of my best story ideas," says Chen, 52, who runs forty miles a week even when he travels.

Exercise while you explore. Instead of taking a taxi or a tour bus to every museum or statue, transport yourself under your own power. If you're traveling on business, use your workout to experience something of the city besides your hotel conference room. While covering Bill Clinton in India, Ed Chen saw even more than he had bargained for: "I saw every kind of animal — donkeys, sheep, goats, camels, elephants," Chen recalls. "I was running along, not paying attention, and there was this cobra rising out of a basket. This was not a run when I was lost in thought."

Pare down your workout schedule. Some exercise is much, much better than none at all. In fact, workout novices can make significant fitness gains with just fifteen 10-minute sessions of exercise each week, according to recent research. (See Chapter 5.) If you're an exercise veteran, research suggests, you can drastically shorten your workouts for up to four months and lose very little fitness. The key is to maintain your intensity. Do one set of strength exercises instead of three, but lift enough weight to fatigue your muscles. Swim fewer yards but push hard. This strategy worked for Portland, Oregon, writer Sarah Bowen Shea on a three-month trip around the world. Shea rarely had time to seek out a pool, let alone fit in 50-minute workouts. But when she did swim, she made the most of her laps. "I'd warm up for ten minutes and then do some really intense intervals," recalls Bowen Shea, 35, who maintained virtually all her fitness. "I'd use my sports watch to make sure I was matching my usual times."

Prioritize. If your schedule is so booked that there's simply no room for exercise, make room. Skip that last antique shop, art gallery, or black-jack table. Forgo happy hour with your coworkers. You'll feel better for it — physically and mentally. "When I don't exercise, my stress level goes up and it becomes apparent in my business dealings," says Pam Kanthor of Dallas, 41, director of IT support for the Dave and Busters restaurant chain. Kanthor, who travels fourteen weeks a year to new restaurant locations, often works sixteen hours a day. Still, she finds the time to exercise most mornings at her hotel gym. "If I don't exercise, I'm not as polite as I should be," Kanthor says. "The people around me are very happy when I work out."

Obstacle 2: "I'm too jet-lagged."

Jet lag, an astute person once observed, is nature's way of making you look like your passport photo. The more time zones you cross, the more confused your body's inner clock becomes and the more you resemble that wretched picture. You know the symptoms: disorientation, fatigue, insomnia, headaches, queasiness, poor concentration, bowel irregularity, and the feeling that you are reliving your worst college hangover. Jet lag is even more severe when you fly east than when you fly west. On an eastbound flight, your day gets shortened, which runs counter to your body's natural inclination to extend the day. (Think about how much easier it is to stay up late than wake up early.)

Jet lag can be a pretty darned good excuse not to exercise. It's a real phenomenon that can last several days, and you shouldn't ignore it. Otherwise, you may end up like former president George Bush, who once threw up on the prime minister of Japan soon after arriving in Tokyo. "The president was playing tennis with the emperor when he should have been sleeping," says former Harvard University professor Martin Moore-Ede, M.D., Ph.D., CEO of Circadian Rhythms (circadian.com), a Boston-based consulting company that helps businesses run round-the-clock workforces. "He went overboard and it all caught up with him."

The following tips, compiled with the help of Dr. Moore-Ede, will help you minimize jet lag. The sooner your body adjusts to your new time zone, the sooner you can manage a regular work — and workout — schedule.

Schedule your flights carefully. Aim to arrive at your destination in the early evening (local time), if possible. By the time you get settled and eat dinner, it will almost be time to go to bed. Since you'll already be tired from the very act of traveling, you shouldn't have much trouble getting to sleep at the proper time, even if your internal clock is out of whack. By contrast, if you arrive in the morning you may be tempted to crash right away, a scenario that can leave you feeling wide awake at midnight local time.

Start your trip well rested. Stress and sleep deprivation will only exacerbate crankiness, fatigue, and other jet-lag symptoms, so plan ahead. Pack early to avoid a 2 A.M. search for the outlet converter that will enable you to blow-dry your hair in Greece. Don't wait until the last minute to pay your bills, cancel your newspaper, put your mail on hold, and buy lithium camera batteries.

Time your sleep correctly. As soon as you board, set your watch to the time zone of your destination, and plan your sleeping schedule accordingly. If it's bedtime where you're headed, make every effort to sleep on the plane. Use a blindfold, earplugs, a pillow, a blanket. Wear comfortable clothing and take off your shoes. If it's daytime at your destination, try to stay awake. Rent a DVD player and a few movies at the airport so you won't run out of entertainment on the plane. Read a book, listen to music, indulge the woman next to you when she starts bragging about her grandchildren.

Drink plenty of fluids. Would you spend five hours in Death Valley drinking nothing but coffee and cocktails? We think not. Yet plenty of people dehydrate themselves on plane flights, where the humidity level is often below 10 percent — lower than in most of the world's deserts. The consequences aren't minor: Your cells start drawing water out of your blood, your blood becomes thicker, and your heart must work harder to circulate blood to your muscles. Your muscles get shortchanged on oxygen and nutrients, and you lose energy and concentration. Bring water on board, and drink one liter for every six hours of flight time. Sure, it's annoying to keep climbing over your fellow passengers to get to the lavatory, but, as the next item indicates, moving around is another great strategy for countering jet lag.

Exercise. While you're flying, take frequent walks in the aisles, and do the stretches in Chapter 13. The exercise will increase blood flow to your muscles and make your body feel less tight and cramped. Stretching and walking during a flight or train ride — or stopping to move around during a long car or bus trip — also is important for preventing travel-related thrombosis, the formation of dangerous blood clots due to excessive sitting. In extreme cases, the clots can travel to your lungs, heart, or brain, causing seizure and death. Rare as this condition may be, it's still pretty good incentive to take periodic strolls down the aisle.

When you arrive at your destination, go for a moderate workout. "Exercise helps my body overcome that spaced-out feeling you get after spending seven hours in a pressurized vessel," says Continental Airlines pilot Joe Payne, 48, who crosses five time zones on his Hawaii-to-Guam route. "And fresh air is huge for recovering from jet lag. You feel like you're connected with the earth again. It's the only thing that makes me feel like I'm on top of my game." However, if you're so wiped out upon arrival that you barely know where you are, a better strategy is to nap before your workout. Payne takes the sleep-before-exercise approach on his Hawaii-to-Houston route, which lands him in Houston at 7:30 A.M. — 3:30 in the morning Hawaii time. Postponing your workout is also a good idea if you arrive close to bedtime; the increase in heart rate and body temperature is likely to disrupt your sleep.

Use light to your advantage. Research shows that bright light can help reset your internal clock — and you don't have to fly to the Caribbean to benefit. There's enough light on a cloudy day in Dublin to do the trick. Be sure to time your light exposure carefully. Bright light in the morning will help adjust your internal clock forward, so you can fall asleep earlier and wake up earlier in the days ahead. Light exposure in the evening will turn your clock back, enabling you to stay up later.

Obstacle 3: "I'm too tired."

Traveling from New York to Miami — or even to Santiago, Chile — won't leave you jet-lagged because you haven't crossed any time zones. But, of course, either journey can wipe you out, as can long car trips, business meetings, or sightseeing itineraries that involve visiting nine French castles in two days. Here's how to feel less tired on the road.

Get a better night's sleep. Studies show that, jet-lagged or not, travelers have more trouble getting to sleep and staying asleep than they do at home; they also spend less time in the restorative stages of sleep. Why? Dr. Moore-Ede chalks it up to the anxiety, stress, fatigue, and excitement of travel. But restless nights aren't a given. To maximize your snooze time, choose a hotel with lightproof curtains, the kind that will make noon in Samoa seem like midnight in the Siberian winter. "It takes only a small amount of light to wake you up," Dr. Moore-Ede cautions. Request a quiet room, away from traffic, and don't bring your worries to bed. For the two hours before you turn in, empty your mind with unchallenging activities — meditating, easy reading, listening to music. Avoid alcohol during those prebedtime hours as well. Although booze may help you fall sleep, it may actually disrupt your slumber about two hours later, a phenomenon that sleep experts call rebound insomnia.

Take a nap. Napping can curb exhaustion the same way a snack can take the edge off hunger. But timing is everything. Keep your siestas to less than 30 minutes, Dr. Moore-Ede advises, and avoid even a short snooze within 4 to 5 hours of your local bedtime. L.A. *Times* correspondent Ed Chen uses the napping strategy when he's bouncing from city to city to city. "I'll give up an hour of sleep overnight in order to get in a run, and then I'll catch up throughout the day with mini naps on the bus or plane," Chen says. "It works for me. I can almost fall asleep at will." The federal government recognizes the restorative power of napping, requiring three-person pilot crews on long-haul flights so that pilots can take turns catching a few winks.

Ease up on your workouts. We know we said earlier that intensity is the key to maintaining fitness on the road, but if you're exhausted, it doesn't make sense to run yourself into the ground. Both sleep deprivation and overtraining can suppress the immune system, increasing your risk of catching an infection. So go easy today — or skip your workout altogether — get a good night's sleep, and crank it up tomorrow. That's the strategy favored by Continental Airlines pilot Mike Brown, who flies the world's longest commercial route, the 15-hour-and-40-minute Newark–Hong Kong flight, which covers twelve time zones. "If I'm tired I don't push it," says Brown, 43, who lifts weights and uses cardio machines on the road. "I don't think that's productive. A lot of times the intensity of my workout isn't nearly as good as it is at home, but that's okay. The important thing is just to get it in."

Realize that exercise actually <u>gives</u> you energy. After a long car trip, bus excursion, or snail's-pace museum tour, have you ever said to yourself, "I can't believe I'm so tired from doing *nothing*"? It may seem counterintuitive, but sitting idle can leave you more exhausted than exercising. That's because your body is meant to move.

When it doesn't, your blood doesn't circulate as efficiently and your lungs don't suck in as much oxygen — the gas that fuels your body's engine. Meanwhile, your muscles fatigue while working overtime to hold you in that rigid position.

Exercise, on the other hand, literally wakes up your body. More blood flows to your muscles, making your body feel more fluid and less stiff, and your brain releases chemicals that make you feel happier and more alert. As tired as Chris Lehane was during the 2000 presidential campaign, he suspects he'd have been even more zonked if he hadn't jogged almost daily. "Even when we were getting five hours of sleep," Lehane says, "it was worth it to lose one of those hours just to get the energy back." Of course, choosing exercise over sleep is generally not a sound idea, given the hazards of sleep deprivation. But over the course of your trip, you'll feel much less lethargic if you make time for exercise than if you never break a sweat.

Obstacle 4: "There's no equipment."

Sure, not every hotel has a gym. And some establishments may take great liberties with the term *fitness center.* You might find a weight machine with fraying cables or an exercise bike that wobbles. Still, equipment problems are a minor obstacle to working out on the road. Here's what to do when the machinery isn't up to par.

Bring your own gadgets. Sex therapist Diana Wiley travels with a rubber exercise tube as insurance against inadequate hotel weight equipment. "You can do your whole strength routine in fifteen minutes while you watch CNN," she says. To cover herself on the cardio front, Wiley purchased a jump rope that was offered as part of the minibar assortment in a Palo Alto, California, hotel room. (See Chapter 11 for a tubing workout and Chapter 6 for jump-rope routines.)

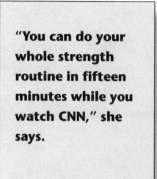

"You can do your whole strength routine in fifteen minutes while you watch CNN," she says.

If packing light isn't a necessity, you can get even more creative. When Lynyrd Skynyrd drummer Michael Cartellone, 38, tours with the band, he brings along a folding steel contraption for dips and pushups. "The hotel luggage guys are always thinking, What the hell is this thing?" Cartellone says. Rock band tour manager Chuck Hull, 48, who has traveled with Lynyrd Skynyrd, Joe Cocker, and Peter Frampton, among others, always brings his road bike, which can be dismantled to fit into a 26-by-26-by-10-inch case. "At hotels, the gym hours usually don't work for me," Hull says. "Plus the equipment is so inconsistent. I don't like to rely on anyone but myself."

Exercise without equipment. You don't need a dip machine, a bench press, or a squat rack for a decent strength workout. A bed, a desk, and a chair can suffice, at least for a while. Chapter 12 shows you how to work almost all of your major muscle groups in your hotel room. If you venture outside, you can expand your repertoire. Canadian Guido Schnelzer, who travels around North America working odd jobs, has no trouble staying in shape without formal workout machinery. If he drives by a park, he'll stop and do pull-ups on the monkey bars and pushups on a picnic table. He also does dips on the tailgate of his truck, propping his feet up on milk crates. "It's all about making the most of what you have," Schnelzer says.

In the cardio department, it's easy to stay fit without a treadmill or bike. Chapter 6 shows you how to burn calories and boost your heart rate using your hotel steps. Climbing real stairs can make a stair-climbing machine seem like a stroll in the park. Plus, in most places, you can head out the front lobby and put one foot in front of the other.

Adjust your workout. Some people stay wedded to their routines longer than they stay in their marriages. They do the exact same exercises in the exact same order for years on end. But you need to be flexible on the road. If your hotel has a seated chest press rather than the horizontal version you're used to, give the new contraption a try (with a light weight, until you figure out how much poundage you can handle). If the hotel has no chest equipment at all, get on the floor and do some pushups. If traveling forces you out of your rut, that's a good thing. When you stick with the same routine endlessly, you tend to plateau. Working your muscles at different angles will only make you stronger.

Obstacle 5: "I don't have the motivation."

Even if you aren't jet-lagged, haven't overbooked your schedule, and have plenty of fine equipment at hand, sometimes you just don't feel like exercising. You start drumming up really dubious excuses not to work out, like "I'd better practice my presentation for the forty-second time" or "I must go back to the Mount Rushmore gift shop to look at the coffee mugs." Here's how to combat plain old inertia.

Exercise with a friend or coworker. Some people enjoy exercising alone and have no trouble getting motivated for a solo effort. Pam Kanthor isn't one of them. She's much more likely to use her hotel gym if she meets up with her Dave and Busters coworkers. "I travel with people who work out," she says, "so we're always encouraging one another. It's a constant conversation: 'Do you want to work out?' 'What time are you working out?'" If you're traveling alone, make a pact with a friend at home and motivate each other via e-mail. Some fitness trainers e-mail their clients on the road to help them stay motivated.

Track your workouts. Whether you keep a formal workout diary (see Chapter 2) or jot a few notes in your Palm Pilot, recording your exercise sessions — "30-min. jog, Phoenix" or "hotel room strength wkt., Denver" — will spur you on. It's always inspiring to see your accomplishments right there in black and white. L.A. *Times* correspondent Ed Chen notes his running mileage in his calendar. When the weather is lousy or he's feeling lazy, he coerces himself into exercising by writing down his mileage before he goes running. "That way, if I didn't go, I'd have to cross it out," Chen says.

Keep your workouts short. If you climb your hotel stairs for ten minutes or do one set of each exercise on a multistation weight machine, how bored can you really get? Plus, if you squeeze in short workouts here and there, you won't feel as if your workouts are cutting into your day.

Consider the consequences of skipping exercise. "To me, exercise is a necessary evil for not gaining weight when I fly," says pilot Mike Brown. "I just think about the price I'll pay for not working out." There's also a price to be paid for letting your muscles atrophy and your cardiovascular fitness vanish: Resuming your workouts can hurt. If you put a bit of effort into maintaining your fitness on the road, you won't have to deal with sore or achy muscles when you get home, and you won't find yourself gasping for breath during a 30-minute treadmill workout that used to be a breeze.

Finally, if you just can't muster up the motivation to work out, think about the best reason of all: your health. Before his bout with colon cancer, Cleveland trucker Ray Kasicki never gave exercise much consideration. "I'd lie down in bed and turn on the TV and that was it," says Kasicki, 54, who drives up to seventy hours a week hauling everything from onions to aluminum coils to bags of clay. These days Kasicki does sit-ups and squats in the cab of his truck, and a couple times a week he'll walk laps around a truck stop. "You appreciate life more after chemo and radiation," Kasicki says. "If I want to be here, it's worth the extra effort."

Clearly, life on the road poses some extraordinary workout obstacles, yet plenty of travelers rise to the occasion. Those who are most successful seem to share one important attribute: adaptability. Wherever you go, relax your expectations and exercise your creativity as well as your muscles. From Guido Schnelzer's inventive use of picnic benches to the mind game Ed Chen plays with his day planner, there's no shortage of strategies that seasoned travelers invent to stay fit.

Of course, not every strategy mentioned in this chapter will work for you. Pam Kanthor thrives on exercising with her Dave and Busters coworkers, but Ray Kasicki wouldn't be caught dead power-walking around a parking lot alongside another trucker. "It wouldn't be good for my image," he jokes. You might find it impossible to concentrate on reading material while you're pedaling a stationary bike. Or you may find it to be no problem at all. Every time you travel, experiment with new approaches.

As you hit on the strategies that suit you best, you may find, to your surprise, that squeezing in exercise isn't such a struggle. Your workouts may become less of an obligation and more of a treat — or at least a habit. Over his sixteen-year career as a pilot, Joe Payne has relied on his hotel gym workouts to give his life on the road some structure. "When your head is on a different pillow four or five nights in a row, it helps to have rituals — and working out is one of them," Payne says. "It provides some semblance of normalcy to your life."

2

Fitting Fitness into Your Suitcase

To keep up an exercise program on the road, you need determination, realistic expectations, and a willingness to adapt. But the right mindset will get you only so far. You also need the right stuff in your suitcase. This doesn't mean you have to pack an entire sporting goods store in your expandable, convertible backpack. Toting around heavy luggage is not a recommended form of exercise. However, a few well-chosen items can mean the difference between staying in shape and letting your fitness fade away.

Some of the products included in this chapter are exercise gadgets; they'll guarantee you a great cardio or strength workout even if you're nowhere near a health club. Other gizmos recommended here are motivational tools. They'll spur you on when you get bored or impatient and feel like throwing in that hotel gym towel. The remaining items simply make exercise more comfortable or convenient.

All of the products are light and reasonably priced, and most take up less space than a travel hair dryer. Review this chapter well before your next trip so you have ample time to make your purchases. Run down the list again while you pack. If you forget to bring shampoo or a toothbrush on your trip, you can rectify the situation with a call to housekeeping or a trip to the market. But you're not likely to find an emergency supply of inflatable kickboards at the concierge desk or a tubing door attachment at the nearest 7-Eleven. The more

> **A few well-chosen items can mean the difference between staying in shape and letting your fitness fade away.**

tricks you have in your travel bag, the less tempted you'll be to skip your workouts.

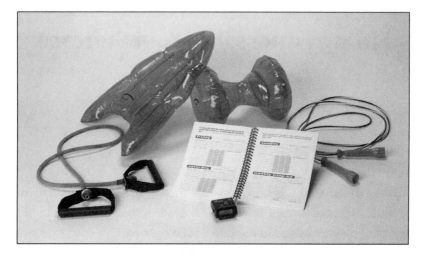

Workout Gadgets

An Exercise Tube

A rubber tube is the most useful strength-training gadget you can pack. It may not look like a very formidable piece of exercise equipment, but just try it. With thick enough tubing, even veteran weightlifters can get in a challenging workout.

The exercises shown in Chapter 11 use a tube with handles. These tubes cost $6 to $12 and come in five to ten thicknesses, depending on the brand. The thicker the tube, the more resistance it offers. You may want to pack two tubes, as some exercises require more resistance than others. If you don't have room for a tube with handles — if, say, you're on a camping trip and every square inch counts — bring a flat band. A band isn't as comfortable to hold but takes up less space than a package of beef jerky.

If you'll be staying in a hotel, consider bringing a door attachment. For a few extra bucks, you can mimic the cable pulley exercises you do at the gym, vastly expanding your exercise repertoire. Two excellent investments are the Fit for Travel Kit (spriproducts.com) and the Lifeline Tote Gym (bodytrends.com). Both cost about $30 and include two tubes, a door attachment, an exercise manual, and a video, all of which fit into a carrying case the size of a makeup bag. Other tube and band products are sold through performbetter.com.

A Jump Rope

Pack a jump rope and you'll never be denied a great cardio workout. A rope is ideal when you can't get to a gym and it's too dark, unsafe, or unpleasant to go walking or jogging. Chapter 6 includes jump-rope workouts you can do in your hotel room or outside.

We recommend a "speed rope," a thin, lightweight rope made of soft plastic. The handles are compact and the rope weighs almost nothing. A speed rope doesn't turn as smoothly as some heavier ropes, but it's more portable and won't do as much damage if it happens to hit a lamp. You can buy one at a sporting goods store for $5 to $10.

Choose a jump rope that fits your body. A rope that's too short will catch your feet frequently; one that's too long will be difficult to get around a full turn without losing speed under your feet. To find the right length, stand on the center of the rope with your feet together, and pull the handles toward your shoulders. You should have a few inches between the end of the handles and your armpits.

An Inflatable Kickboard and Pull Buoy

The only swim essentials are a cap, goggles, and — in most cases, anyway — a swimsuit. However, your workouts will be more challenging and enjoyable with a kickboard and a pull buoy, a gadget that you stick between your legs to keep them stationary while you focus on working your upper body. The $12 Zura Swim Travel Kit includes a nifty inflatable kickboard and pull buoy; each takes about 90 seconds to blow up. You also get a mesh carrying pouch. Check out zura.com.

Motivational Tools

A Pedometer

Sometimes the incentive to exercise comes from getting credit for your effort. You might be more motivated to take a walk during your airport layover if you know how much ground you've covered. A pedometer — a beeper-sized gadget you clip onto your waistband — measures walking or running distance in both steps and miles. You program in the length of your stride, and the device senses every step you take. Some models also record your pace, total time spent exercising, and calories burned. (Consider the calorie numbers a gross estimate.) Wear your pedometer when you're sightseeing, too, and set specific distance goals for the day or the week.

How accurate is a pedometer? To find out, we tested six models on a half-mile course. Four of them were fairly accurate, calculating the distance to be between .45 and .48 miles. (The discrepancy may have been partly due to human error in measuring stride length.) These models were also very reliable; each pedometer recorded virtually the exact same distance in each of four trials. However, some of the models were maddeningly difficult to program, partly because of instruction manuals written with a less-than-fluent grasp of English. The two models we liked best were the Bodytronics Q25 Electronic Pedometer for $21.95 and the Part Ultrak 275 Electronic Calorie Pedometer for $26. These and other pedometers are sold through bodytronics.com.

A Workout Log

Did you jog for 30 minutes in Detroit on Tuesday, or was it in Des Moines on Monday? Or wait — maybe you lifted weights in Des Moines and ran in Dubuque. When you're traveling, it's tough enough to keep track of what time zone and city you're in; remembering how many times you've exercised in the last week is next to impossible. Yet tracking your workouts can be a valuable motivator. If you flip through your log and notice you've exercised just once in the last week, you may be inspired to spend 15 minutes of quality time with your jump rope.

Make notes in your day planner or in an exercise diary designed for recording cardio, strength, and stretching workouts. The back of this book features log pages to help you get the hang of tracking your exercise sessions. At the beginning of each week, list concrete goals for the coming days. "Walk 1/2 hour 3 times and do 2 weight workouts" is more useful than "Exercise when possible." For each session, record your time and/or distance — whether you walked for 2.7 miles at the airport (according to your pedometer) or pedaled for 20 minutes on the hotel bike. Track your strength workouts in as much or as little detail as you desire. You could record your sets and repetitions or simply note "Tubing routine."

Recording all these details may seem like a hassle, but compared to the tabulations required for business travel — car mileage, hotel costs, restaurant expenses — tracking exercise is a breeze. Plus, your log (unlike that delinquent expense reimbursement check) offers instant gratification.

A Portable CD Player/Radio

It's pretty tough to stay motivated on the treadmill when your hotel gym's TV is tuned to C-SPAN or a Turkish-language cooking show — or the gym has no TV at all. Listening to your own music can inspire you to keep sweating and offer a welcome comfort zone in a setting that's otherwise disorienting.

Several electronics manufacturers offer portable compact disc players designed for exercise. Panasonic's ShockWave CD Jogger and Aiwa's Cross Trainer feature an antishock memory system designed to provide skip-free CD listening for nearly anything short of high-impact aerobics. These models spin discs faster than normal while the audio data is digitally recorded. If the CD does skip, the system plays the music from memory until the tracking problem is fixed. Priced at about $180, the players are also water-resistant and promise to run up to 20 hours on two AA batteries.

Investments for Comfort and Convenience

A Water Bottle or Hydration Pack

Drinking plenty of water can help you recover from jet lag, minimize travel fatigue, stave off weight gain (by making you feel more full), and improve your workout stamina. So keep a water bottle handy at all times — on the plane, in the car, at the gym, in your hotel room, on your tour of the Egyptian pyramids or Universal Studios.

If you plan to exercise outdoors, whether you hike, bike, or ski, consider investing in a hydration pack such as a Camelbak. It's an insulated pouch that you fill with water and wear on your shoulders like a backpack or around your waist. To drink, you bite down on the end of a tube that hangs over your shoulder. Drinking water is so convenient that you don't even realize you're doing it. Plus, your hands are free to hold your ski poles, carry your portable radio, or brace yourself if you fall. (Hydration packs are great for climbing hotel stairs, too.) Most hydration packs have pockets for stashing snacks, keys, maps, cell phones, identification, and money. Some are large enough to double as a backpack, so you can take it hiking or stuff it with workout clothes on your way to a local gym. Check out camelbak.com for a look at the numerous models.

Quick-dry Clothing

Opening a suitcase to find soggy, stinky workout clothing will not inspire you to hit the treadmill. Our advice in three words: Don't bring cotton. Instead choose synthetic tights, shorts, tops, sports bras, and socks that will dry quickly after you wash them in your hotel sink. Lightweight fabrics such as Patagonia's Capilene, Nike's Dri-FIT, and CoolMax can almost be shaken dry. (And even if they're still damp when you're ready to work out, they won't feel uncomfortable.) Acrylic socks with CoolMax woven into them dry especially well and retain their shape.

If you're traveling in cold climates and need an insulating layer, fleece is ideal. It weighs almost nothing and keeps you warm even if you get caught hiking in a downpour or get sprayed by sprinklers. A black fleece vest is practically essential travel gear if you plan to exercise outdoors. It's great for layering and stylish enough for everyday wear.

Comfortable Athletic Shoes

This should go without saying, but bring sturdy, well-cushioned athletic shoes, and wear them on your travel days. You might not look very fashionable, but if you get trapped for five hours between flights, you can at least burn some calories to kill the time. Walking distances in dress shoes not only is uncomfortable, but also can lead to all sorts of foot, knee, and hip injuries. If you need to wear business attire upon your arrival, pack your dress shoes in your carry-on bag.

A Lock

You may be able to drum up some decent excuses not to work out, but "my stuff might get stolen" isn't one of them. Some gyms will lend or rent you a lock, but don't count on this service. Keep a lock in your bag at all times.

A Gym Bag

Try to bring carry-on luggage, such as a small backpack, that can double as a gym bag. If that's not possible, pack a small, bona fide gym bag. This way you can conveniently tote around your swim gear, towel, or workout clothes if you end up at a gym or pool that's not in your hotel.

Weightlifting Gloves

Gloves may seem like an extraneous item — something only Mr. Universe contestants would pack. But they take up virtually no space, make weightlifting much more comfortable, and protect your hands from developing calluses. The weight equipment at your hotel gym might not have the padded or contoured grips of your gym at home. If the handles are too slippery or too rough, you may be tempted to abandon your workout.

3

Finding Gyms, Trails, and Pools on the Road

There's an awful lot to hunt down when you travel. If you're not searching for the best local sushi bar or breakfast nook, then you're trying to find the subway, the freeway, or the Internet café — or the mate to your blue fleece glove. How can you deal with locating a place to work out?

Actually, it's not such a daunting task. You almost have to venture into a Tanzanian game park to be able to say, with any legitimacy, that you couldn't find a dumbbell to lift or a safe route to run. Locating a place to sweat simply takes a bit of initiative — picking up the phone, chatting with the concierge, logging on to the Web — and, at times, a sense of adventure.

A sense of humor helps, too. When David Negus was on business in the Philippines, a cab driver delivered him to a building marked HEALTH CLUB. After paying an entrance fee, Negus was led to the exercise room, which consisted of two weight bars and a few light weight plates. "I quickly realized this served as a cover for a massage parlor and brothel," says Negus, 45, deputy controller for Population Services International, a Washington, D.C.–based nonprofit organization. "The weights were covered with spider webs and dust." Negus chose to forgo the massage and work out his biceps and triceps.

Whether you're traveling in Southeast Asia or southeast Ohio, your search for a bona fide health club will probably be more fruitful than Negus's. This chapter gives you the resources to find gyms, jogging routes, and swimming pools just about anywhere your itinerary takes you.

Finding a Gym

There are nearly 17,000 health clubs in the United States; chances are, you're not far from one of them. Of course, you're more likely to find a top-notch facility if you're staying at an upscale hotel or in a big city than at a motel or in a small town (this is especially true internationally). But well-equipped gyms are now popping up in modestly priced hotels, rural areas, even airport terminals. Here's a look at the various gym choices you're likely to encounter on your travels.

Scouting Out Hotel Fitness Centers

"Hotel gym" used to be an oxymoron, but the percentage of U.S. hotels with fitness facilities has skyrocketed, from 36 percent to 56 percent in the last decade. Among hotels with 250 rooms or more, 79 percent have gyms, according to the American Hotel and Motel Association. The figure is 70 percent for hotels with 150 to 249 rooms. Hotel gyms aren't as prevalent internationally, but most high-end establishments offer fitness centers, many that rival the best North American gyms. These days you can find hotel clubs in many countries — even places as far off the beaten path as Madagascar — where they may not have existed five years ago.

> "Hotel gym" used to be an oxymoron, but the percentage of U.S. hotels with fitness facilities has skyrocketed, from 36 percent to 56 percent in the last decade.

The amenities at hotel gyms vary widely. At midpriced establishments you might find one treadmill, one stairclimber, one stationary bike, and a small array of dumbbells, or none at all. Some hotels, fearful of liability, won't put free weights in unsupervised gyms, instead offering weight machines, which are safer but less versatile. Many of these machines are of high quality; others have deteriorating cables, torn seat padding, and substandard engineering that could end up separating you from your shoulder. Larger resort hotels may have more amenities than your gym at home, including rock climbing, yoga, Pilates, and tai chi classes. Many high-end hotels also offer personal trainers (typically for at least $50 to $75 an hour). Almost all hotel gyms are free to guests, although some with spa facilities do charge guests to use the exercise equipment, even if they're not using the whirlpool and sauna.

Some establishments, including certain Hilton, Hyatt, and Ritz-Carlton Hotels, will even transform your room into a gym, delivering a stationary bike, yoga videos, jogging trail maps, fitness magazines, and exercise tubing. Some hotels charge extra for these room-service gyms; others don't.

When booking your hotel, ask very specific questions about the equipment. "Cardio machines" can mean elliptical trainers hooked up to the Internet or flimsy stairsteppers without any electronic feedback. "Weight facilities" can mean a complete line of shiny, freestanding machines or one small, rusty contraption that requires an engineering degree to operate. Also ask about the hours. Some hotel gyms are open twenty-four hours to anyone with a room key; others are closed overnight.

If you haven't booked a room in advance, ask to tour the facilities before you hand over your credit card. Some hotels have been known to exaggerate or omit key information, like the fact that the hotel's fitness center is closed for renovations. When Carolyn Cade of Minneapolis inquired at the front desk about workout facilities at her hotel in China, she was sent to the second floor. She discovered that the gym was indeed open for business, but not the sort of business she was looking for. "When I looked in, I saw exercise equipment as well as a lot of businessmen and six women in various stage of undress," recalls Cade.

Some hotels don't have fitness centers on-site but have agreements with clubs in walking distance, which you can use free or for $5 to $10. This can be a great deal; you may have to walk a block or two, but you get much more extensive facilities than most hotel gyms offer.

Exercise Facilities at the Major Hotel Chains

You're heading to St. Louis: Should you book a room at the Hyatt, the Marriott, or the Days Inn? The following list, summarizing the policies of many major hotel chains, may help you decide. (Some large chains were unable to provide fitness information.) The facilities at each location may vary, so be sure to call ahead. Note: "Weight machines" typically refers to multi-gyms rather than a line of individual machines.

Clarion

(800) 252-7466, clarionhotels.com

Fitness facilities: All (not all are on-site; some hotels have agreements with local clubs)

Type of equipment: Cardio machines; weight info N/A

Comfort Inn

(800) 221-2222, comfortinn.com

Fitness facilities: Varies from location to location

Pools: Varies

Type of equipment: Cardio machines; some have multi-gyms

Country Inn and Suites

(800) 456-4000, countryinns.com

Fitness facilities: 30 to 40 percent; required for new hotels with 50+ rooms

Pools: 95 percent

Type of equipment: All fitness centers have cardio machines; only some have weights

Crowne Plaza

(800) 227-6963, crowneplaza.com

Fitness facilities: All

Pools: Most

Type of equipment: Cardio machines, weight machines

Days Inn

(800) 325-2525, daysinn.com

Fitness facilities: 16 percent

Pools: 84 percent

Type of equipment: Cardio machines, weight machines

Doubletree

(800) 222-8733, doubletreehotels.com

Fitness facilities: 90 percent

Pools: 90 percent

Type of equipment: Varies

Four Seasons

(800) 332-3442, fourseasons.com

Fitness facilities: All

Pools: 95 percent

Type of equipment: All fitness centers have cardio machines and weight machines and/or free weights, 50

percent have studio classes, 90 percent have certified trainers

Hilton

(800) 445-8667, hilton.com

Fitness facilities: All

Pools: All

Type of equipment: Varies

Holiday Inn

(800) 465-4329, basshotels.com

Fitness facilities: 98 percent

Type of equipment: Varies

Homewood Suites

(800) 225-5466, homewood-suites.com

Fitness facilities: All

Type of equipment: Cardio machines; weight equipment varies

Hyatt

(888) 468-6839, hyatt.com

Fitness facilities: All (not all on-site; some hotels have agreements with a nearby gym)

Pools: 75 percent

Type of equipment: Most fitness centers have cardio machines and free weights

Marriott

(800) 228-9290, marriott.com

Fitness facilities: 95 percent

Pools: 95 percent

Type of equipment: Cardio machines, free weights, and weight machines

Ramada

(800) 272-6232, ramada.com

Fitness facilities: Varies

Pools: Varies

Type of equipment: Varies

Red Lion

(800) 733-5466, hilton.com

Fitness facilities: All

Pools: All

Type of equipment: Cardio machines and weight machines; some have free weights

Ritz-Carlton

(800) 241-3333, ritzcarlton.com

Fitness facilities: All

Pools: 80 percent

Type of equipment: All fitness centers have cardio machines and weight machines and/or free weights

Sheraton Hotels and Resorts
(800) 325-3535, starwood.com
Fitness facilities: All
Pools: 95 percent
Type of equipment: Cardio machines, weight machines

Summerfield Suites
(800) 996-3426, wyndham.com
Fitness facilities: All
Pools: All (some closed in winter)
Type of equipment: Cardio machines

Westin Hotels and Resorts
(800) 228-3000, westin.com

Fitness facilities: All (95 percent with on-site facilities)
Pools: All
Type of equipment: Cardio machines, weight equipment

Wingate Inn Hotels
(800) 228-1000, wingateinns.com
Fitness facilities: All
Type of equipment: Cardio machines, weight machines

Wyndham Hotels
(800) 996-3426, wyndham.com
Fitness facilities: 75 percent
Pools: 50 percent
Type of equipment: Cardio machines and both free weights and weight machines

Tracking Down a Local Club

If your hotel doesn't have a gym or its facilities are inadequate, you can probably find a club nearby, although typically you'll need a car, cab fare, or reliable instructions for getting there via public transportation. Not only will you feel better for having made the effort, but if you mingle with the locals, you may score some tips on the area's best bars and restaurants. You may also want to look for a local club in the middle of a long driving day on a road trip. A moderate workout, followed by a shower in the club, can get you back on the highway feeling energized and refreshed.

Even if your hotel has a decent gym, tracking down a local club can be worthwhile as a cultural diversion. Ask around Lincoln, Nebraska, and you may find a gym frequented by local heroes, some very chiseled Cornhusker football players. Visit any upscale club in Los Angeles and you'll witness a cultural phenomenon that may make you glad you're only visiting the city: gym members shouting into their cell phones while pumping away on the stairclimber. (Warning: Avoid asking anyone wearing a cell phone to spot you on the bench press. If the phone rings while you have 150 pounds of steel teetering above your chest, you can guess where your spotter's priorities will reside.)

Exercising at clubs abroad offers even more opportunity for educational and entertaining experiences. Make some inquiries in Micronesia, and you might find the tin shack on Yap island where locals lift heavy barbells while chewing betel nut, a mild narcotic that turns their teeth red, permanently. Do some legwork in Chad and you may locate a gym plastered with old Arnold Schwarzenegger posters where members lift homemade dumbbells — made of steel bars and cement blocks — while seventies disco music blares from a cassette player. Pick a gym at random in Cairns, Australia, and you're likely to encounter the most shocking cultural oddity of all, at least where gyms are concerned: out-and-out friendliness. If you accidentally sit on a machine someone was about to use, you might actually hear "No worries, mate!"

Finding a local club may also be worthwhile for the classes. Whether you take group cycling, tai chi, or step aerobics, a class can be an excellent way to lift flagging motivation. With an instructor to inspire you (even in a foreign language) and fellow class members to keep up with, you'll probably push yourself harder than you would on your own — just like at home. You may also get a few chuckles from the experience. While traveling in France, Miami trainer Adita Yrizarry took an aerobics class accompanied by some really raunchy American rap music. Although neither the instructor nor the students spoke English, they had memorized the lyrics and sang them loudly and with great passion. "They had huge smiles on their faces, but they had no idea what they were singing," Yrizarry says. "I've never laughed so much."

A class can also make you feel more relaxed in an unfamiliar city. After landing in Stuttgart, Germany, Los Angeles photographer Stephanie Waisler went straight to a Spinning class. "Getting on a Spinning bike always feels exactly the same, no matter what the music or the language," says Waisler, 34, who has taken group cycling classes while traveling on business in several European countries. "It's comforting when you're feeling disoriented." However, Waisler didn't feel quite so at home outside of the Spinning room, where gym members were smoking and drinking beer at small tables in the snack bar area.

What's the best way to find a local club? Seek information from several sources. Here are some ideas.

Ask the concierge. But don't take his or her word as gospel. The guy at the front desk may know as much about exercise as you do about Civil War trivia. Also, in countries where exercise is less popular, concierges may not be familiar with the local workout options.

Look in the phone book under "health clubs" and "gyms." Bring your list to the concierge to find out which clubs are closest. Then call the clubs for information about hours, equipment, directions, and fees. Most gyms (other than Bally's clubs and many YMCAs) offer day passes to nonmembers, but fees can vary drastically — from $5 to more than $25 at some swanky New York City clubs.

Ask the locals. If you're at the supermarket and spot someone whose biceps are bursting out of his or her shirt, ask for a gym recommendation. If you're at a bar, ask the bouncer. Don't be shy; fit people love to talk about exercising, especially if you start the conversation with "Excuse me, but you look like you work out . . ."

Use the Internet. Check out both healthclubs.com and nutricise.com (their databases overlap quite a bit). Both sites let you search clubs according to facilities offered — such as group cycling classes or child care — but call the gym to double-check the accuracy of this information. Here's a closer look at the two sites.

- Healthclubs.com: This site helps you locate clubs that are members of IHRSA, the International Health, Racquet and Sportsclub Association, a Boston-based trade group with about 6,000 member clubs in the United States and abroad. Pros: A nifty map that shows you where the clubs are in relation to one another, plus a link for point-to-point driving directions. Also, club listings in more than 50 foreign countries, from Argentina to Qatar. Cons: The site includes only IHRSA clubs, excluding about 60 percent of clubs nationwide.

- Nutricise.com: This comprehensive fitness and nutrition site features a gym locator in its "Healthy Living Tools" section. Pros: The database includes a whopping 10,000 clubs, with phone numbers and addresses. Also, you can narrow your search to within a certain proximity of the Zip Code — for instance, within five miles of Santa Monica, California 90402. Cons: No maps or foreign gyms.

A Look at National Gym Chains

If you frequently travel to major cities, you may want to join a national chain, so you have free access to member clubs or franchises throughout the country. Just make sure that the chain actually has clubs in the cities you visit and that they are conveniently located.

If you belong to a club affiliated with IHRSA, the International Health and Racquet Sportsclub Association, another option is to join the association's Passport program. If your home club is an IHRSA member, ask for a Passport sticker, which gives you access to more than 3,600 clubs worldwide, some of which aren't usually open to travelers. Some, but not all, of the clubs offer a day-pass discount to Passport members. Check out healthclubs.com to find out which clubs participate in the Passport program.

Here's a look at the dominant chains and their travel policies.

24-Hour Fitness (24hourfitness.com)

This chain also has more than 300 clubs nationwide, along with several dozen worldwide. Log onto the company's Web site to find a club near you, whether you're in Atlanta, Cleveland, or Oslo, Norway. If you're in a foreign country, you can use any 24-Hour Fitness for up to 30 days at no cost. If you're not a member, you typically can buy a daily guest pass.

Bally Total Fitness (ballyfitness.com)

The Bally site can lead you to any of the chain's 300-plus clubs nationwide. Most, but not all, membership levels give you free access. If you're not a member, look for another gym; Bally clubs do not regularly offer day passes to nonmembers. You may be able to work out once or twice as a guest, but only if you're willing to take a tour and endure a sales pitch. Bally day passes are geared toward attracting new members, not accommodating travelers who don't intend to join a Bally club.

Gold's Gym (goldsgym.com)

Gold's isn't a chain but rather a network of franchises with more than 500 locations in 26 countries. If you're a Gold's member, you'll typically need a travel pass from your home club to work out for free (or at a discount) at other Gold's clubs. All Gold's gyms allow day passes to nonmembers, typically charging $10 to $15.

YMCA (ymca.net)

The country's 2,400 YMCAs operate autonomously, and policies differ from one Y to the next, although a membership at one can almost always get you admitted to any other location. At many locations, you can exercise for free at off-peak times, but you may have to pay during rush hour. Some clubs charge visiting members half the guest fee and restrict the number of yearly visits allowed. Some clubs don't allow nonmember guests at all. To find the nearest Y in the United States, call (888) 333-YMCA or go to ymca.net, which also has links to international YMCAs. To find a Y in Canada, go to ymca.ca.

Airport Gyms: Working Out During Your Layover

On a short layover, your best exercise option is to stow your carry-on in a locker and power-walk around the airport. However, if you have a few hours to kill, a real workout may be just the ticket — to fight boredom, the lure of Cinnabon, or the urge to drop $70 on a hip-swiveling Elvis clock that says "Welcome to Columbus."

A handful of airports have gyms right inside a terminal or at a hotel attached to the airport. They have showers, towel service, toiletries, massage, and lockers big enough for your monster carry-on. A few sell or rent workout wear. The table on pages 36–39 lists workout facilities in or close to major North American airports.

A Rubdown at the Airport

By the time you unfold your body from its in-flight position and drag your weary self and your carry-on bags off the plane, you pretty much feel like the dregs. Your neck and shoulders are in knots. Your head is clogged from the stale air. Your bag has created a semipermanent dent in your shoulder. What you need is a massage. If you're lucky, you've landed at an airport that offers one right there in the terminal. (If you're smart, you won't get so engrossed in the rubdown that you miss your boarding call and nearly miss your flight, not an unprecedented occurrence.)

Most airport massage bars offer a chair massage for about $1 a minute, with a minimum of 10 to 20 minutes. Usually that's enough time to work out the kinks and restore your circulation so you can walk out of the airport — or onto your next flight — feeling more human.

Perhaps one day massage bars will be as ubiquitous at airports as Starbucks. In the meantime, here's a list of those that were in business at press time. Hours may vary.

Anchorage: Ted Stevens International Airport
The Right Spot
(907) 786-0847, cpleitez@webtv.net
Near the food court and Starbucks
Mon.–Sat., 12 am–9 pm

Boston: Logan International Airport
A Relaxed Attitude
(617) 567-0933
Terminal B, American Airlines side,
   upper level
Hours vary

Chicago: O'Hare International Airport
Backrub Hub (Spa Nation)
(773) 601-0630
Terminal 3
Daily 9 am–9 pm

Denver: Denver International Airport
A Massage Inc.
(303) 342-7485, www.amassageinc.com
Main Terminal West, Level 6 (ticketing),
   near the post office
Daily 7:30 am–9:30 pm

Nashville: Nashville International Airport
Massage Bar, Inc.
relax@massagebar.com,
   www.massagebar.com

A/B Concourse entrance, just beyond the
   security checkpoint
Sun.–Fri. 11 am–7 pm

Orlando: Orlando International Airport
Profiles Express Salon Massage
(407) 825-6485
3d floor, B side, near Bank of America
Mon. 12 pm–8 pm,
   Tues. 2 pm–7 pm,
   Wed. 12 pm–8 pm,
   Thurs. and Fri. 12 pm–7 pm,
   Sat. 12 pm–8 pm, Sun. 1 pm–8 pm

Pittsburgh: Pittsburgh International Airport
Touch and Go
(412) 472-3323,
   BillTouchngo@netscape.net
United/TWA Airlines Concourse
Daily 8 am–8 pm

Seattle: Seattle-Tacoma International Airport
Massage Bar, Inc.
www.massagebar.com
Concourse C entrance, just beyond
   security checkpoint and at the North
   Satellite between Gates N-16 and N-1
Concourse C: Daily 9 am–9 pm
   North Satellite: Sun.–Fri. 7 am–8 pm,
   Sat. 7 am–6 pm

Finding Running Routes

Going for a walk or a jog is a great way to burn calories, relieve stress, inhale some fresh air, and see the sights. If there's no gym around — or you're positively allergic to indoor exercise — it may be the only option. But if you're in unfamiliar territory, ask the concierge at your hotel about the neighborhood's safety before you set off to explore. While jogging in Chad, David Negus accidentally ran into five armed men guarding a palace. "They all pointed guns at me, and I backed up really slowly, trying to show them I had no weapons," Negus says.

Cristina Acosta of Bend, Oregon, nearly encountered danger of a

Where to Exercise on Your Next Airport Layover

Airport	Fitness Center Name	Address
Atlanta: Hartsfield Atlanta International	Perimeter Summit Health Club	4000 Summit Blvd.
Baltimore: Washington International	American Athletic Club	3916 S. Hanover St.
Boston: Logan International	Hilton Hotel	Attached to airport by enclosed skybridge
Calgary: Calgary International	World Health Club	2525 36th St. NE
Charlotte: Douglas International	Gold's Gym	6010 Fairview Rd.
Chicago: Midway	Al's Gym	5301 W. 65th St. #708
Chicago: O'Hare International	Hilton Chicago O'Hare Airport	Adjacent to terminal 2, via pedestrian tunnel
Cincinnati: Northern Kentucky International	Fit Works Fitness & Sports	7541 Mall Rd., Florence, KY
Cleveland: Hopkins International	Bally Total Fitness	3600 Park East
Dallas: Ft. Worth International	Irving Fitness Center	297 West Langrove Rd., Irving, TX
Denver: Denver International	World Gym Fitness Center	1515 E. Colfax Ave., Aurora, CO
Fort Lauderdale: Hollywood International	Gold's Gym	3120 Oakwood Blvd., Hollywood, FL
Honolulu: Honolulu International	24 Hour Fitness	98199 Kamehameha Hwy., Aiea, HI
Houston: William P. Hobby	24 Hour Fitness	12260 Gulf Hwy.
Indianapolis: Indianapolis International	Indy Fitness	6355 Westhaven Dr.
Kansas City: Kansas City International	Just Total Fitness	8114 NW Prairie View Rd.
Las Vegas: McCarran International	24 Hour Fitness	In Airport (main terminal)
Los Angeles: Los Angeles International	24 Hour Fitness at the Hilton	On lower level of LA Airport Hilton
Memphis: Memphis International	Fitness Plus	2598 E. Corporate Ave.
Miami: Miami International	Miami International Airport Hotel	Concourse E
Minneapolis: St. Paul International	Appletree Fitness Center at Holiday Inn	3 Appletree Sq., Bloomington, MN
Montreal: Dorval	Nautilus Plus	8305 Cote De Lisse
Nashville: Nashville International	Gold's Gym	2311 Murfreesboro Pike
New York: John F. Kennedy International	Cross Island Sports & Fitness	219–10 S. Conduit Ave., Springfield Gardens, NY
Oakland: Oakland International	Integrated Fitness Group	833 Island Dr. #D
Orange County, CA: John Wayne	Club Met-RX	140 E. 17th St. #B, Costa Mesa, CA

Distance	Hours	Phone Number
20–25 min	5:30am–8:00pm M–F, 10–2 Sa	(404) 256-6527
10 min	8am–10pm M–T, 8–9 F, 9–4 Sa	(410) 355-1494
5 min	5:30am–11pm M–F, 6:30–10 Sa–Su	(617) 568-6700
15 min	5am–11pm M–F, 8–6 Sa–Su	(403) 590-9250
10 min	5am–10pm M–F, 8–6 Sa, 12–6 Su	(704) 554-1010
5 min	6am–10pm M–T, 6–9 F, 9–6 Sa, 9–3 Su	(708) 563-9334
	5:30am–11pm M–T, 5:30–10 F, 6–10 Sa–Su	(773) 686-8000
10 min	6am–11pm M–T, 8–8 Sa–Su	(859) 282-0600
10 min	5:30am–11pm M–T, 5:30–10 F, 8–8 Sa–Su	(216) 267-3500
5 min	24 Hours	(972) 257-0221
15 min	7am–10pm M–Sa	(303) 344-4413
7 min	5am–12pm M–T, 5–10 F, 8–8 Sa–Su	(954) 927-3481
15 min	24 hours	(808) 486-2424
10 min	24 hours, 7 days	(713) 943-2220
10 min	5am–10pm M–T, 5–9 F, 7–9 Sa, 9–5 Su	(317) 532-0344
5 min	5am–10pm M–F, 8–7 Sa, 10–6 Su	(816) 505-0900
		(702) 261-3971
	24 hours	(310) 410-9909
5 min	6am–7pm M–F, 8:30–12:30 Sa	(901) 345-1036
	6am–10pm M–Sa	(305) 871-4100
5 min	6am–10pm M–F, 8–7 Sa, 10–6 Su	(952) 854-3691
5 min	6:30am–10pm M–F, 9–4 Sa–Su	(514) 739-2289
5 min	24 hours M–F, 8–9 Sa, 9–9 Su	(615) 366-1063
10 min	8am–10pm M–T, 8–8 F, 9–5 Sa, 10–2 Su	(718) 528-7592
5 min	5:30am–9pm M–F, 8–6 Sa–Su	(510) 864-2030
10 min	5am–10pm M–F, 7–7 Sa–Su	(949) 645-1677

Airport	Fitness Center Name	Address
Orlando: Orlando International	World Gym	1900 S. Semoran Blvd.
Philadelphia: Philadelphia International	Old City Ironworks	141 N. 3rd Street
Phoenix: Sky Harbor International	Phoenix Suns Athletic	230 S. 3rd St.
Portland, OR: Portland International	Nelson's Nautilus	8333 NE Russell St.
Raleigh: Raleigh–Durham International	Rex Wellness Center	4200 Lake Boone Trail
Salt Lake City: Salt Lake City International	Apple Fitness	324 S. State St. #100
San Antonio: San Antonio International	Olympic Gym	8611 N. Newbraunfels Ave.
San Diego: San Diego International	Sheraton East Tower	1380 Harbor Island Dr.
San Francisco: San Francisco International	Gold's Gym	2301 Market St.
San Jose: San Jose International	Gold's Gym	600 Meridian Ave.
Seattle: Seattle–Tacoma International	Powerhouse Gym	15233 Pacific Hwy. South
St. Louis: St. Louis International	St. Louis Workout	212 N. Kings Hwy.
Tampa: Tampa International	Beach Park Health Club	3637 S. Manhattan Ave.
Toronto: Lester B. Pearson International	Sporting Club	10 Carlson Court, Etobical, ON
Washington, D.C.: Ronald Reagan	Old Town Sports & Health	209 Madison St.

different sort while staying at an upscale Orlando hotel with canals running through the grounds. "I just thought I'd go through a run on this sandy road at the edge of the complex," Acosta recalls. "When I walked through the lobby in my running clothes and waved to the concierge, she said, 'Wait, you can't go running around here. Don't you know about the alligators?'"

Even if you're not likely to be assassinated by armed guards or devoured by reptiles, you may be at risk for getting hopelessly lost if you don't have a route in mind — or on paper — before you head out. Fitness consultant Liz Neporent has had to call a cab more than once to rescue her from a run gone awry. "I always think I'm going in a straight line, but I make turns without realizing it," says Neporent, who travels internationally setting up corporate fitness centers. Once, while on business in Los Angeles, Neporent accidentally roamed into a residential neighborhood without foot traffic or pay phones. "I finally knocked

Distance	Hours	Phone Number
5 min	5am–11pm M–T, 5–10 F, 8–8 Sa–Su	(407) 249-5506
10 min	5am–11pm M–T, 5–10 F, 7–8 Sa, 8–8 Su	(215) 627-7002
15 min	5am–8:30pm M–F, 8–2 Sa	(602) 379-7500
5 min	5am–11pm M–F, 8–8 Sa–Su	(503) 254-7710
15 min	6:45am–9:30pm M–T, 6:45–8 F, 8:30–6 Sa, 1–6 Su	(919) 784-1371
15 min	4:30am–11:30pm M–F, 7–9 Sa, 8–8 Su	(801)521-9400
5 min	5am–10pm M–F, 8–6 Sa–Su	(210) 829-5040
5 min	6am–10pm M–Sa	(619) 291-2900
20 min	5am–12pm M–T, 5–11 F, 7–9 Sa, 7–8 Su	(415) 626-4488
5 min	5am–12pm M–F, 6–9 Sa–Su	(408) 279-6441
3 min	24 hours	(206) 433-1555
15 min	5:30am–10pm M–T, 5:30–9 F, 8–6 Sa–Su	(314) 633-3020
10 min	9am–9pm M–F, 9–4 Sa	(813) 839-4444
5 min	5:45am–11pm M–F, 9–6 Sa–Su	(416) 674-5313
5 min	5:45am–10pm M–F, 8–7 Sa	(703) 548-6822

on some door and this woman peeks through the chain and barks, 'What do you want?' Instead of letting me in, she handed me a cell phone through the letter slot."

Neporent was luckier than *Los Angeles Times* White House correspondent Ed Chen, who once got lost in the dense fog in Orlando — the same morning he was supposed to cover a speech by Bill Clinton. Waving furiously to motorists from alongside the highway, he tried in vain to hitch a ride to his hotel. Ultimately Chen did find his way back, but not before jogging for nearly two and a half hours. He arrived just as Clinton's motorcade was pulling away from the hotel. "I jumped in a cab," Chen says, "and just as I walked into the hall where he was speaking, they were starting 'Hail to the Chief.' "

Unless you have the time or fitness to jog sixteen miles on your outings, take precautions: When you walk or jog in a new area, always carry the phone number and address of your hotel, along with identification and, if possible, a cell phone. A fanny pack or hydration pack with pockets (see Chapter 2) is an excellent way to carry all this stuff while keeping your hands free.

Here are some tips for finding running or walking routes. As with gyms, it's best to get your information from more than one source.

Ask the concierge. At large hotels, staff members are usually equipped to answer this question and may even have jogging maps. (Some Ritz-Carlton hotels have a "jogger's station" set up at the main entrance each morning, offering chilled towels, bottled water, and route maps.) However, you may end up with a concierge who doesn't quite realize the difference between driving a particular route in a car and covering that same distance on foot. Beware if the concierge says something like, "Make a right and not that far down you'll see a park. I don't know, it might be a little uphill . . ."

Call a running store. Look in the phone book for specialty stores that sell running shoes and gear. These stores are usually operated by avid runners, who can suggest the perfect route, whether it's a six-mile dirt trail or a two-mile stroll through town.

Go to runnersworld.com. The "On the Road" section, listed under "News and Reference," links you to articles that have appeared in *Runner's World* magazine describing the running options in more than 80 cities. You'll find directions to dirt trails and city routes, as well as phone numbers and Web sites for local running clubs. Local running stores also are listed. Just beware that some of these articles may be outdated.

Locating a Pool

If you're a swimmer, you may get frustrated with hotel pools. Some are so short that you'd get dizzy doing flip turns. Others are oddly shaped. "That can be like swimming in milk because you can't perceive where you are," says Portland, Oregon, writer Sarah Bowen Shea, who travels frequently on assignment. "I'm good at swimming straight, but not that good." You may also have to contend with screaming children, over- or underheated water, and mega-doses of hair-frying, skin-drying chlorine. That's when you need to find a real pool.

In most cities, it's not that difficult to locate one, assuming you have transportation and enough time. One great option is a YMCA membership, which gives you access to Y pools all over North America and in many countries abroad. In addition to looking in the phone book and asking your hotel staff, try these two Web sites:

> **Beware if the concierge says something like, "Make a right and not that far down you'll see a park. I don't know, it might be a little uphill . . ."**

Swimmer's Guide Online. swimmersguide.com. This remarkable site can lead you to more than 9,000 full-size pools in the United States and more than 90 other countries. With a few clicks, you can find the address, phone number, cost, length, and water temperature of all the pools in any town, city, or region. Another plus: This site contains links to masters (adult) swim clubs, so you can join a local workout. You can also find a list of nearby hotels, invaluable information if you're an avid swimmer who wants to choose a hotel for its proximity to a pool.

A Scientific Guide to Lap Pools Worldwide. kilmartin.com/pools. This site, created by New York City stand-up comic Laurie Kilmartin, rates only 110 pools nationwide, but it's so darned funny that it's worth visiting even if you don't know how to dog-paddle. Kilmartin, who has traveled as much as forty weeks a year during her career, assigns each pool a letter grade, lists the amenities (pace clocks, kickboards, lane lines), and offers amusing commentary. Of the 90-degree YWCA Pool in Augusta, Georgia, Kilmartin writes: "Severe dehydration set in after two minutes and the water fountain was tucked away in the locker room. Every three hundred yards or so I had to crawl out of the deep end like an American P. O.W. on the last mile of the Bataan Death March."

4

Eating on the Fly

Cruise the highways of southern Kansas and you may drive past a giant wooden sign offering nutritional advice from the heartland: EAT BEEF, KEEP SLIM. Therein lies the challenge of eating healthfully on the road.

Wherever you go — a steakhouse in the Midwest, a hotel coffee shop, a fast-food joint at the airport — you encounter food, and lots of it, that's not exactly friendly to your waistline (or your arteries). Not that beef can't be a part of a nutritious diet; any food can, in moderation. But when you dine out for every meal, you're not likely to consume the leanest cuts of meat, the most vitamin-packed salads, or the most fiber-rich breakfast cereals. And when you're killing time at airports, attending cocktail parties with clients, and frequenting popular restaurants at your vacation destination, you end up eating more than you do at home. Even if you exercise regularly on the road, you can easily return home carrying a few extra pounds.

The good news is that you have more healthy choices than ever at many chain restaurants and airport food courts. Still, it takes vigilance to control your calorie intake — and to consume a meal or snack with any semblance of nutritional value. Denny's offers a nutritious Oatmeal 'N Fixins breakfast (535 calories, 3 grams of saturated fat, 7 grams of fiber), but it's right there on the menu with the Cinnamon Swirl Slam (1,105 calories, 26 grams of saturated fat, 2 grams of fiber). That Starbucks cinnamon raisin bagel (320 calories, no fat) is sitting in the same display case as the chocolate croissant (480 calories, 11 grams of saturated fat). As you ponder your options, you're probably battling that mysterious condition that often afflicts travelers — the one that causes you to think, Hey, I'm on a trip! The calories don't really count!

Making good food choices requires more than resolve. You also need nutritional savvy, and you need to do your homework, as the best options aren't always obvious. The Burger King Big Fish Sandwich might appear to be a more healthful selection than a Whopper with cheese — hey, it's fish! — but it actually has more calories (710, compared to 620) and the same amount of saturated fat (a whopping 14 grams). A typical restaurant order of spaghetti with meatballs has twice the calories — 1,160 — of the typical serving of rib-eye steak. Who'd have guessed?

This chapter will help you order wisely when you travel, whether you're at the airport, on the plane, at a fast-food restaurant, or at a steak joint in the heartland. Don't worry: You don't have to travel on wheat bagels and carrot sticks to avoid coming home heavier. You can dine at Big Bubba's BBQ without turning into Big Bubba himself.

Nutrition by the Numbers

A 6-inch meatball sandwich at Subway contains 10 grams of saturated fat. Is that a lot or a little? The sub also contains 3 grams of fiber. Is that substantial or not? To make use of the nutrition information in this chapter, on package labels, and on restaurant Web sites, it helps to have an understanding of nutrition basics. You needn't spend your trip counting calories and fat grams, but you can make better choices if you have a rough idea of your nutrient needs. This section will help you put the numbers in context.

Calories. How much of a dent will a bear claw (600 calories) make in your daily calorie budget? A registered dietitian can give you a fairly precise number based on your weight, muscle mass, activity level, and other factors. But you can use the following formula to generate a ballpark figure for your calorie needs. Let's say you weigh 150 pounds.

Step 1: Translate your weight into kilograms by dividing it by 2.2. You weigh 68 kg.

Step 2: Multiply your weight in kilograms by 24 to arrive at your resting metabolism, the number of calories you burn daily simply to stay alive. Your resting metabolism is about 1,636 calories.

Step 3: Multiply your resting metabolism by an "activity factor." Use 1.2 if you spent all day on the plane. Use 1.5 for light activity and 1.7 for a moderately active day. Use 2.0 if you're on a bike tour in the Italian Alps. If you spend the day buckled to your plane seat, that bear claw would account for nearly one-third of your 1,960 daily calorie needs.

> **As you ponder your options, you're probably battling that mysterious condition that often afflicts travelers — the one that causes you to think, Hey, I'm on a trip! The calories don't really count!**

Fat. Most major health and nutrition organizations recommend getting no more than 30 to 35 percent of your total calories from fat — about 66 to 77 fat grams on a 2,000-calorie-per-day eating plan. However, this is a somewhat arbitrary recommendation, as not all fats are created equal.

Unsaturated fats, such as those found in olive oil, avocados, and nuts, contain the same 9 calories per gram as saturated fats, but they are essential to good health. Not only is unsaturated fat important for keeping HDL cholesterol levels healthy, but it's also essential for the absorption of several vitamins. If the vast majority of your fat intake comes from unsaturated fat, it appears that your health will not be compromised by exceeding the 30 to 35 percent recommendation (as long as your total calorie intake is not excessive).

The real culprit is saturated fat, the artery-clogging, cholesterol-raising kind found primarily in animal products, such as beef, chicken, milk, ice cream, and cheese. Health organizations recommend limiting saturated fat to 10 percent of total calories, but preferably 7 percent. If you eat 2,000 calories a day, that means you should limit your saturated fat intake to about 16 to 22 grams a day. To put this number into perspective: a Starbucks Classic Coffee Cake contains 18 grams of saturated fat.

Also watch out for trans fats, found in fried foods and processed baked goods. These fats raise blood cholesterol levels just as much as saturated fats do, but they're not as well known because the government does not require trans fat numbers to be listed on food labels. (This rule is likely to change.) Trans fats are created through hydrogenation, a process that turns liquid oils into solids such as margarine and shortening. Hydrogenation makes pie crusts flakier and french fries crisper. You can get an idea of how prevalent trans fat is by consulting burgerking.com, the only major fast-food Web site to offer trans fat information. Trans fat accounts for nearly half the harmful fat in a large order of BK onion rings, adding 7 grams to the 6 listed in the saturated-fat column; in other words, fast-food fries are twice as harmful to your arteries as you might think. If you eat fried foods, doughnuts, Danish, cookies, or crackers, limit your portions and dip well below those 16 daily grams of saturated fat to make room for trans fats.

Protein. If you pay attention to protein numbers, you'll see why a 6-inch roast beef sandwich at Subway may be a better lunch choice than the 6-inch Veggie Delite sandwich. True, the veggie sub has 60 fewer calories, but it also has 10 fewer grams of protein (and no additional fiber). Protein takes longer to digest than carbohydrate, so if you choose meals and snacks that combine the two nutrients, you'll stay satisfied longer than if you eat a meal that's primarily carbohydrate. Experts recommend getting about 15 percent of your daily calories from protein. (That's about 75 grams of protein on a 2,000-calorie diet. One gram of protein contains 4 calories.) The Veggie Delite gets only 7 percent of its calories from protein, compared to 27 percent for the roast beef sub. When you feel satisfied after a meal, you're less likely to indulge in junk food two hours later.

Fiber. Fiber may be the toughest major nutrient to come by when you're on the road. It's plentiful in fruits, veggies, and whole grains — none of which are particularly abundant at airports and fast-food restaurants. High-fiber foods help protect against heart disease, diabetes, and, possibly, cancers of the breast, pancreas, stomach, and colon. They also help you control your weight because they tend to be filling and low in fat. Although experts recommend eating 25 to 35 grams of fiber a day, Americans typically eat just half that amount. When you're traveling, a good way to rack up fiber is to eat oatmeal (3 grams of fiber per single-serving packet) for breakfast and beans wherever you can (a Taco Bell bean burrito contains 7 grams of fiber).

Eating at the Airport

When you're at the airport, food is often transformed from nourishment to entertainment. Sure, you can kill time by reading the newspaper, shopping for overpriced sweatshirts, maybe checking your e-mail. But eating always seems to be the main attraction, especially when your flight is delayed or you're in the midst of a stressful journey. What's more comforting: an airline employee's apology for your lost luggage or a freshly baked cinnamon roll?

If you search hard enough, you can eat nutritiously at any airport in North America. However, you'll have to look harder at some airports than others. A recent survey by the Physicians Committee for Responsible Medicine rated San Francisco International best among the country's top-ten busiest airports. Twenty-four of twenty-five restaurants there offered at least one low-fat, high-fiber, cholesterol-free meal. At other airports, only one-third of the restaurants served nutritious fare.

"For many travelers, the airport is where good eating habits start to slide," says St. Louis dietitian Ellie Zografakis, who counsels many frequent flyers. "So survey the airport before you make any rash decisions." Zografakis offers the following tips so that you don't have to loosen your belt when you board your next flight.

Don't arrive at the airport hungry. Eat a full-fledged meal before you go to the airport because you probably won't make the best choices once you're there. Hunger makes you more impulsive and less able to focus. With the scent of Cinnabon wafting through the terminal, what ravenous person is going to lunge for the apple and turkey sandwich at the deli counter? If you weren't able to eat earlier, make a concerted effort to consume an airport meal that includes both protein and carbohydrate. That chocolate frozen yogurt may take the edge off your hunger temporarily, but it won't hold you over for four hours.

Assess whether you're truly hungry. Were you lured to the keilbasa cart because you're homesick for your native Pittsburgh? Are you scooping malted milk balls out of the candy bins because you're bored? If your stomach isn't telling you loudly and clearly that you need to eat, stroll past the food court and find other ways to amuse yourself. Read a magazine, call a friend, play Travel Scrabble with a companion, compose e-mail on your laptop, do some people-watching. Or, better yet, lock up your carry-on bag and go for a walk.

Avoid alcohol. Just because there's a bar in your terminal doesn't mean you have to park yourself there. The calories in alcohol go down way too easily. Plus, booze makes you less inhibited and stimulates your appetite, so you're likely to keep digging into that huge bowl of buttered popcorn sitting in front of you. Also, pre-flight drinking will contribute to the dehydration that's so common while flying (see Chapter 1). Apparently, not too many travelers heed this advice: According to a survey by the National Sleep Foundation, about 25 percent of business travelers say they drink more alcohol on the road than they do at home.

> What's more comforting: an airline employee's apology for your lost luggage or a freshly baked cinnamon roll?

Think ahead. Before you get in line at Starbucks, consider the day in front of you. If you're going to eat lunch on the plane and meet clients for drinks and dinner when you arrive, the calories you consume at the airport are extraneous. If you grab a Grande Low-fat Mocha and a lemon bar before you board, you're consuming nearly 900 calories — almost half the calories you may need for the entire day.

Airport Snack Foods: The Good, the Bad, and the Astonishingly High in Fat

Which has more calories: a jelly-filled doughnut at Dunkin' Donuts or a low-fat cranberry peach muffin at Starbucks? An Auntie Anne's Mocha Dutch Ice or a Starbucks Grande Mocha Frappuccino? Most of us would probably choose our snacks more carefully if the nutrition information were posted in bold type at the cash register. Unfortunately, it's usually not, although most major chains do post nutritional information on their Web sites and may have brochures available at some locations. Here are some tips to help you make decisions at three popular airport snack venues.

Starbucks

If you're craving a fancy coffee drink, the pecking order is as follows, from fewest calories to most. (All are "grande" size with nonfat milk.) Cappuccino (110), Latte (160), Frappuccino (270), Mocha (320). On the pastry front: The bagels are fat-free with about 300 calories, but unpalatable, if you ask us. Muffins range from 420 to 530 calories with 8 to 12 grams of saturated fat. The low-fat muffins are a better deal: only slightly lower in calories (360 to 400) but at least free of saturated fat.

Those giant cookies range from 400 to 450 calories and from 4 grams of saturated fat (ginger molasses) to 11 (oatmeal raisin and chocolate chip). The scones weigh in at 500 calories and 8 grams of saturated fat. The worst offenders: Classic Coffee Cake (629 calories, 18 grams saturated fat), buttermilk cinnamon roll (709 calories, 12 grams saturated fat), and maple oat nut scone (556 calories, 16 grams saturated fat). In terms of calories and disease-promoting fat, all are comparable to or worse than a Big Mac.

Dunkin' Donuts

As indulgences go, an Old-Fashioned Cake Donut sounds like a decent option: only 250 calories and 3 grams of saturated fat. Ah, but there's that hidden artery-clogging fat: The trans fat in one of these doughnuts more than doubles the damage that its saturated fat inflicts on your heart, according to the Center for Science in the Public Interest, a nonprofit organization that has analyzed the saturated-fat content of many restaurant menu items. Dunkin' Donuts bagels actually contain more calories than the doughnuts — about 340 on average — but they have negligible fat, 11 grams of protein, and some fiber (3 grams in the cinnamon raisin bagel and 4 grams in the wheat bagel). The muffins are not a great choice: 500 to 590 calories. If you're counting calories and craving a doughnut, go for a sugar-coated raised (170 calories) or glazed (180).

Auntie Anne's Pretzels

Pretzel-wise, Auntie Anne is generally looking out for your health. The pretzels aren't low-calorie — mostly in the 300 range without butter and about 450 with butter. However, they typically contain about 4 grams of saturated fat with butter (virtually none without butter), making them a much better option than a muffin. They have one-third more calories than a typical doughnut, but at least contain some fiber. The whole-wheat pretzel has 7 grams of fiber, as much as a bowl of bran cereal. Even the Glazin' Raisin pretzel contains 4 grams of fiber. However, if you want a blended coffee drink, march over to Starbucks for a Frappuccino. Auntie Anne's Mocha Dutch Ice contains 570 calories (about 300 more than a Grande Frappuccino), including a whopping 12.5 grams of saturated fat.

In-Flight Meals: A Nutritional Mystery

Sautéed sea bass with sun-dried tomato sauce, lamb medallions with mint jus, seafood bisque in a sourdough bread bowl — airline food is no longer the oxymoron it once was. But while in-flight meals have become tastier in recent years, have they become any more healthful? Does the typical airplane dinner contain 800 calories or 1,800?

It's hard to tell, because nutritional information for plane food generally is not available. If you go to an airline's Web site, you'll typically find a listing of special meals, such as low-fat, low-cholesterol, vegetarian, and so on. But you won't find any nutritional data about standard meals, and even the special-meal information is very limited. For instance, the United Airlines site (ual.com) lists the foods prohibited and allowed in its low-calorie menus, but the site does not reveal how many calories are in a low-calorie meal!

In search of more complete information, particularly for regular meals, we contacted eight major airlines, requesting menus with recipes, nutritional breakdowns for economy and first-class meals, and/or general nutritional guidelines. We came up nearly empty.

Most of the airlines were happy to tell us about their "incredible food service" and their "interesting, exciting, and innovative" new menu items, but only Southwest — which serves snacks instead of meals — provided actual numbers for anything but special meals. The other airlines said they didn't have the information (because menus are constantly changing) or didn't have the time to collect it.

We weren't the only ones who had trouble tracking down nutritional breakdowns for in-flight fare. Nutricise.com, a fitness and nutrition Web site, made a more extensive attempt, surveying 15 major airlines. In most cases, Nutricise was unable to secure recipes and nutritional information. However, staffers did acquire sample menus, which they analyzed on their own with nutritional software. This task required a lot of guesswork because most of the menus did not include portion sizes, and many did not indicate cooking methods.

The results? Nutricise concluded that the average coach dinner has about 1,054 calories — about half a day's worth. (The site doesn't provide information about saturated fat or fiber.) However, there was a very wide range, from 534 calories on British Airways to 1,643 on Midwest Express. It's impossible to say whether the sample menus provided by the airlines surveyed are typical. It's likely that, as in most restaurants, the calorie counts vary widely from meal to meal.

Don't expect first-class fare to be more nutritious than the food served in economy. In a recent press release, United boasted that its first-class customers can now enjoy Ben and Jerry's ice cream, Mrs. Fields cookies, Eli's Cheesecake, and Godiva chocolates. Nutricise found that one first-class meal on Delta — filet mignon, caesar salad, roasted potatoes, vegetable medley, organic rolls, and an ice cream sundae — contained a whopping 1,829 calories. And that didn't include condiments or beverages!

The bottom line: Just because airline meals are served in small containers on small trays does not mean the calorie counts are small as well. If you're a frequent flyer, it may take extra vigilance to avoid weight gain because you don't have the choices available in a restaurant and the food sits in front of you longer.

One option is to call the airline in advance and order a low-calorie or low-fat special meal. Just make sure you don't overcompensate by splurging at the airport upon your arrival. A United "Heart Smart" breakfast consisting of a high-fiber bagel, fat-free cream cheese, fresh fruit, and orange juice contains 550 calories, certainly a reasonable and nutritious breakfast. But if you supplement this breakfast with a typical airport muffin, you will have doubled the calorie count of your breakfast.

If you don't order a special meal, pay close attention to the food in front of you rather than mindlessly gobbling every item on the tray. Instead of using the whole container of butter, use half and save 50 calories. Ask the flight attendant to remove the dessert so you won't even be tempted. If the plane meal is — or will be — your fourth full meal of the day, skip it. Instead, eat one of the snacks suggested in the next section.

Snacks for the Car and Plane

On a recent road trip in the Midwest, Ellie Zografakis's friends showed up with Twizzlers, fat-free cookies, pretzels, and bags of Sun Chips. "It looked like we were going away for two years," says the dietitian. "But we were driving from Ohio to Chicago. It was a four-hour trip."

Of course, the problem with packing so many snacks is that, out of boredom, you tend to eat them all. When you're traversing central Nevada and the region's only radio station has been interviewing the local JV golf coach for an hour, munching on honey-mustard pretzels becomes a pretty fascinating diversion. When the in-flight entertainment consists of movies you've already seen in the theater and on video, you might scarf down that whole package of Rolo candies without even realizing it.

On the other hand, it's important to be prepared for a snack attack. If you let yourself get too hungry in the car, you may end up ordering the entire left side of the menu for dinner. Become ravenous on the plane, and you'll overindulge at the airport; plus, you'll arrive in a really cranky mood.

Boarding a plane with snacks is particularly important, as 25 percent of flights these days arrive late. It's not unheard of to get stuck on the runway for an hour or two without snack service, in which case you might end up eating the entire box of Icelandic chocolate you bought as a gift for your family. Also, airlines spend considerably less on food than they used to. Whereas you might have gotten a hot lunch in the past, you might get a bagel and a Snickers bar now. And if you're flying Southwest, you'd better be really prepared, as the airline prides itself on cutting costs by serving snacks instead of meals. On a five-hour flight from Providence, Rhode Island, to Phoenix, Arizona, all you'll get is four bread sticks, a cheese cup, a cereal bar, and a cookie — a grand total of 360 calories.

Below are snack suggestions for the car and plane. Zografakis recommends keeping the food out of direct reach — in the trunk, in the overhead bin — so that you can't munch mindlessly. Also, she suggests, bring snacks that aren't your absolute favorite so that you'll eat out of hunger and not just because you enjoy the taste. A bag of Hershey's Kisses is not a good snack idea. Here are some better options.

Energy bars. Luna Bars, Clif Bars, PowerBars — the market is flooded with different brands. Energy bars make great travel snacks because they don't melt or get smushed or stale. But read the labels. Some have as many calories as a candy bar without much nutritional value. Others are fortified with vitamins and minerals and contain a fair amount of fiber and protein, both of which help to keep you satisfied.

Dried fruit. Sure, it's sticky and tough to chew, but that's a good thing, because dried fruit is also fairly high in calories. A 4-ounce bag of dried apricots contains 270 calories. But on the up side: That same bag contains almost 9 grams of fiber. (You get no fiber in a 270-calorie pack of Rolos.)

Nuts. Peanuts, cashews, and other nuts get a bad rap because they're about 70 percent fat, but most of it is the healthy kind of fat. And nuts contain a bit of fiber and varying amounts of vitamins and minerals. Just be sure to bring small, individually wrapped bags, as just 1 ounce of nuts contains some 170 calories.

Pretzels. They're convenient and lower in calories than nuts (about 110 calories per ounce), although pretzels may not satisfy you for long because they are primarily carbohydrate.

Turkey or beef jerky. Jerky may seem like the ultimate junk food, but in reality, most brands are very low in fat and calories and high in protein. A typical 1-ounce pouch of jerky contains 80 calories, 14 grams of protein, and just 1 gram of fat. Chewing it is hard work, so the calories take awhile to add up. Plus, jerky is a nice way to balance high-carb snacks like dried fruit and pretzels.

Baby carrots. You can certainly do worse things to your body than to polish off an entire bag of baby carrots. (One pound of carrots contains just 174 calories.) Nutritious and tasty, these make a great car snack.

Grapes. These, too, are convenient for the car and are a good way to combat a craving for something sweet. One pound of grapes contains about 310 calories and is certainly more satisfying than, say, a 32-ounce, "super-size" soda, which contains about the same number of calories.

Savvy Restaurant Eating

When you shop at the supermarket, you can read the package labels, but when you eat out, you're left to guess how many calories or fat grams are in a particular dish. Some restaurants, such as Denny's and Chili's, offer nutritional information for their light menu items, but virtually no restaurants (outside of fast-food joints) provide calorie counts for their standard menu items.

Sometimes a rough guess will suffice. You can pretty easily deduce that, unless you're a seven-foot NBA center, a 20-ounce porterhouse steak is going to have a lot more calories than your body needs for dinner. You can surmise that any onion-ring appetizer will contain more harmful fat than your arteries can happily accommodate on a regular basis. But what if you want to know more? What's the better choice: The manicotti or the ravioli? The sirloin steak or the rib eye?

One way to find out is to carry around the "Eating Smart Restaurant Guide," published by the Center for Science in the Public Interest (cspinet.org). This handy fold-out card reflects extensive laboratory research and nutritional analysis by CSPI. The guide includes the typical serving size, calories, total fat grams, and the amount of artery-clogging fat (saturated fat plus trans fat) for a variety of restaurant categories, from Chinese to seafood to Mexican. By the way, according to CSPI, that porterhouse contains 1,110 calories, and those onion rings contain 900 calories and 23 grams of saturated fat. The ravioli beats the manicotti and the sirloin beats the rib eye.

Here are some additional tips to help you navigate your way through restaurant menus.

Watch your portions. These days the servings are so enormous that you may get two or three times more than you need. (Ever been to a Claim Jumper?) If possible, split an entree with a friend or order an appetizer portion of the dish. And despite what your mother may have said, you don't need to clean your plate.

Veer off the menu. Most restaurants are willing to accommodate health-conscious patrons, so don't be shy about placing a special order. If your turkey sandwich comes with french fries (590 calories), ask if the cook can round up some fruit or vegetables instead. Fruit and veggies are a great way to fill up and boost your nutrient intake without loading up on calories.

Learn restaurant vocabulary. *Alfredo, au gratin, batter-dipped, béarnaise, breaded, creamy, crispy, parmigiana, tempura* — these are all terms that suggest loads of fat and calories. Words that usually indicate leaner dishes include *grilled, broiled,* and *poached.* You can save a lot of calories by honing your vocabulary. A typical 7-ounce serving of fried clams contains 820 calories, compared to 300 calories for the same size serving of steamed clams.

Ask how dishes are prepared. Even if a dish is described as "broiled," the chef may add butter to keep the poultry or fish moist and shiny. If you learn that an entree is laden with fat, ask for the sauce on the side or ask for another method of preparation. Remember that the restaurant is primarily interested in making your dining experience a delicious one. The chef's agenda may not be your agenda.

> **Unless you're a seven-foot NBA center, a 20-ounce porterhouse steak is going to have a lot more calories than your body needs for dinner.**

Know your meats. You *can* eat beef and stay slim if you choose the right cuts. A typical 12-ounce serving of trimmed sirloin steak contains 390 calories, rib eye contains about 500, and T-bone (typically served in 16-ounce portions) contains 690 calories. Among the worst choices are porterhouse steak (1,100 calories for a typical 20-ounce serving, with 40 grams of artery-clogging fat) and prime rib (1,280 calories and 52 grams of harmful fat in 16 ounces).

Beware of condiments. You don't need sour cream, butter, and cheese on that baked potato, do you? Forgo gravy and cheese sauces, or at least dribble them sparingly on your entree.

Don't assume the word <u>salad</u> is synonymous with "nutritious." At some salad bars it's hard even to locate a vegetable. Instead the tubs are filled with macaroni-and-marshmallow salads, taco salads, and mayo-drenched potato salads. Always go for the darkest greens. Iceberg lettuce is a nutritional zero, and if you plop a couple of tomato slices on top, along with bacon bits and croutons, you're not doing any better. Beans are among the best choices; one-half cup garbanzo beans contains a substantial 8 grams of fiber.

Eat slowly and deliberately. It takes about 20 minutes for the feeling of fullness to register in your brain, so if you wolf down your meal, you'll probably eat more than your body needs to feel satisfied.

Don't deny yourself. If you're craving a burger, order a burger, although preferably without the cheese or mayo. If you ignore your craving and order steamed vegetables instead, you'll probably fantasize about that burger for the rest of the day and end up indulging in a sour cream bacon cheeseburger with fries.

Fast-Food Eating

Question: What's harder to locate than a cheap plane ticket on Thanksgiving weekend? **Answer:** A vegetable on the Burger King menu. The only menu items with at least 5 grams of fiber are king-size orders of fries and onion rings. That fiber comes with a hefty price: nearly enough artery-clogging fat to max out your limit for the entire day.

It's no secret that the growth of the fast-food industry has contributed to the American obesity epidemic (an epidemic now spreading to other nations that are adopting our fast-food habits). Not only are fast-food joints more prevalent than ever before — especially at airports and alongside interstate highways — but they're serving larger portions of their nutritionally void menu items. According to *Fast Food Nation*, Eric Schlosser's exhaustively researched indictment of the fast-food industry, the typical soft drink order at a fast-food restaurant in the 1950s contained about 8 ounces of soda; today a "child-size" order of Coke at McDonald's contains 12 ounces, and a large Coke is 32 ounces, more than 300 calories. An order of supersize fries, which weighs in at 540 calories, is three times larger than what McDonald's sold a generation ago, Schlosser reports.

Even if you don't regularly eat fast food at home, on the road you may, at times, find yourself with few other options. Fortunately, not all fast-food places are as nutritionally challenged as Burger King and McDonald's. Some, including Wendy's and Subway, make it fairly easy to walk away from lunch without feeling like you're oozing grease. Still, you have to order carefully.

Here are some tips for ordering at the major fast-food chains. Keep in mind that the statistics cited don't include trans fat, which typically doubles the amount of harmful fat in fried foods.

Arby's

Many Arby's sandwiches are lower in calories and saturated fat than burger-joint offerings, but don't be fooled by terms such as "Market Fresh." The Market Fresh roast ham and Swiss and the turkey and Swiss sandwiches hover at around 800 calories, twice as much as many of the roast beef sandwiches.

Highlights: The light roast chicken and turkey deluxe sandwiches contain only 260 calories, negligible fat, and substantial amounts of protein. Of course, 260 calories isn't enough for lunch. Combine your sandwich with a baked potato, but instead of having both butter and sour cream (for 500 calories and 15 grams of saturated fat), order one or the other on the side.

Lowlights: The Italian, Philly Beef 'N Swiss, and Roast Beef subs contain about 16 grams of saturated fat, one entire day's worth.

Burger King

Unlike some of its competitors, BK offers no nutritious side dishes. If you're forced to eat at a BK, aim for the smallest portions possible, such as a burger (340 calories). Order everything without mayo, and you'll save about 150 calories.

Highlights: None.

Lowlights: The burgers are scary. The Double Whopper with Cheese weighs in at 1,020 calories, including 32 grams of artery-clogging fat (65 total fat grams). Even a regular Whopper contains 680 calories and 13 grams of disease-promoting fat.

KFC

The Colonel offers what most fast-food joints don't: nutritious side dishes.

Highlights: You get 6 grams of fiber in the BBQ Baked Beans and 4 grams in the corn on the cob. The Tender Roast Sandwich without sauce contains only 270 calories, with 1.5 grams of saturated fat; the sauce adds 80 calories. The potato wedges are at least better than most fries — 280 calories, 4 grams of saturated fat, 5 grams of fiber.

Lowlights: Chunky Chicken Pot Pie weighs in at 770 calories and 13 grams of saturated fat, although you do get 5 grams of fiber.

McDonald's

McDonald's portions are slightly smaller than Burger King's, but you won't find much on the menu with fiber. Also, items that might sound like a good choice — such as the grilled chicken caesar salad, at only 100 calories — may leave you feeling hungry.

Highlights: The Fruit 'N Yogurt Parfait is a decent addition to the menu, at 380 calories, 2 grams of saturated fat, and 10 grams of protein, plus a substantial dose of calcium. (Numbers weren't available, but most yogurts have at least 20 percent of the daily calcium recommendation.) It's certainly a better breakfast choice than the Spanish Omelet Bagel, with 690 calories and 14 grams of saturated fat.

Lowlights: A Big Mac (590 calories) and supersize fries (610 calories) are not good choices. On the breakfast front, don't be tricked by the word *bagel*. The Ham and Cheese Bagel has the same number of calories (550) as the Sausage Biscuit with Egg. The Steak and Egg Cheese Bagel contains a whopping 700 calories and 13 grams of saturated fat.

Subway

Subway is a worthy stop, offering more nutritious choices than most fast-food joints. The company's Web site, subway.com, even offers tips for reducing the calorie and fat content of Subway menu items.

Highlights: The only 6-inch sub that hits 500 calories is the meatball sub. The others, including ham, roast beef, roasted chicken breast, and turkey breast, are generally under 300 calories, although only if you skip the cheese (41 calories) and oil (45 calories). Order your sub with mustard (8 calories) and vinegar (1 calorie) instead. Choose the wheat bread to add an extra gram of fiber. Order baked potato chips instead of fried chips and save 40 calories.

Lowlights: Both the foot-long meatball and Caesar Italian BMT subs contain more than 1,000 calories. Those small, innocent-looking cookies pack a lot of calories, 200 to 220 each, and it's hard to eat just one.

Taco Bell

Taco Bell has one advantage over most fast-food restaurants: its high-fiber bean items.

Highlights: A Pintos 'n Cheese side dish is a reasonable 180 calories, and you score 10 grams of fiber. A tostada (250 calories) contains 11 grams of fiber. A taco salad with salsa — without the shell — gives you 430 calories and 15 grams of fiber. You do get 10 grams of saturated fat, so it's a tradeoff. The chicken burritos are much lower in fiber (about 3 grams) than the bean burritos and beef burritos, and not any lower in calories. On the taco front, look for those served with beans.

Lowlights: Don't be fooled by the word *salad*. The taco salad with the shell contains 850 calories and 14 grams of saturated fat.

Wendy's

Wendy's is the best fast-food choice. The salad bar is loaded with vitamin-packed veggies — such as broccoli, green peppers, and carrots — and it's virtually the only place in fast-food land that you can find a piece of fruit (usually orange and cantaloupe). Choose your salad dressings carefully; blue cheese, French, and caesar have 150 to 180 calories per 2 tablespoons. Go for the reduced-fat or fat-free versions, which add only 30 to 50 calories.

Highlights: Wendy's chili is a great nutritional value: 340 calories (in a large), 3.5 grams of saturated fat, 7 grams of fiber, and 23 grams of protein. Make a meal of it, along with a sour cream and chive baked potato (370 calories, 3 grams of saturated fat, and 7 grams of fiber). The pita sandwiches are generally good choices, topping out at 480 calories, 4 to 6 grams of fiber, and substantial protein.

Lowlights: The Big Bacon Classic contains 580 calories and 12 grams of saturated fat.

Maintaining Your Cardio Fitness

You've got the motivation to exercise, you've packed the right gear, and you've found a place to work out. Now it's time to break a sweat. Part II helps you design the cardiovascular segment of your travel workout program. Cardio exercise, such as walking, stair climbing, and swimming, is one of the three crucial components of any exercise program (the others are strength training and stretching) and the one that generally burns the most calories.

Chapter 5 offers a crash course on cardio basics, explaining how to adapt your home cardio routine to the constraints of your travel itinerary. Among the questions addressed: How often should you exercise on a trip, and how hard should you push yourself? What are the best cardio machines for travelers? Should you tailor your cardio workouts to different climates? Chapter 6 covers your options when outdoor exercise isn't safe and you don't have access to machines. You'll find creative, effective routines for jumping rope and climbing hotel steps, along with calisthenics from your grade school days that you likely forgot all about. Chapter 7 is for people who like to get wet. It explains how to shorten your swim workouts without losing fitness and how to liven up lap swimming so it's not as boring as watching an airline safety video. Chapter 7 also teaches you how to boost your heart rate in a hotel pool that's too short or too oddly shaped for swimming.

5

Cardio 101 for the Traveler

No question about it: Travel qualifies as an endurance sport. Transporting yourself from the airport parking lot to baggage check-in to your departure gate can take the stamina of an athlete — especially if you're schlepping a carry-on bag and hustling to pick up a John Grisham novel before your plane starts to board.

Or let's say you get evicted from a train in the middle of the night in France and have to walk three miles with all your luggage. That's what happened to Brad Kearns, a corporate lifestyle coach at a Silicon Valley software company. A railroad official shook him from a deep slumber at 3 A.M., pointed to his passport, which had expired at midnight, tossed his bags out the door, and demanded that he immediately get off the train, which had made a checkpoint stop at the Belgian border. Kearns then had to drag his suitcases all the way to a commuter train station where passports were not checked. "That was my toughest 5k ever," says Kearns, 36, a former professional triathlete.

You just never know when your fitness is going to come in handy, so it's crucial to keep your heart and lungs in shape if you travel on a regular basis. But traversing airports and train stations isn't the only reason for a traveler to jog, hike, swim, or jump rope. Regular cardio exercise has been shown to reduce stress, a helpful benefit for dealing with surly railroad officials, and improve your sleep, a bonus when you stay in noisy hotels. You can burn several hundred calories in a cardio workout, so this type of exercise is crucial for weight control. Moderate exercise also boosts the immune system, so you may even be less likely to catch a cold on a trip. Being in shape can save you money, too. Instead of catching cabs to local restaurants, shops, and attractions, you can rely on your own two feet.

Cardio fitness is easily gained, but it's also easily lost. The longer you go without exercise, the more you lose and the more time it takes to regain your stamina. This chapter will give you the knowledge to maintain your cardio fitness on a reduced training schedule. You'll also find tips on adapting your workouts to hot and cold climates, along with a chart estimating calories burned during popular cardio activities

The longer you go without exercise, the more you lose and the more time it takes to regain your stamina.

— just so you know how much jogging it takes to burn off that raisin scone you scarfed down at the airport.

Warming Up and Cooling Down

When you're pressed for time, you naturally look for ways to cut corners. If your tour bus to Buckingham Palace leaves in 45 minutes, you may be tempted to hop on your hotel treadmill and run like that *Chariots of Fire* guy for 20 minutes and then dash to the shower. This is not a good idea.

Instead, warm up for at least 5 minutes at an easy pace. Warmer muscles are more flexible and less likely to get injured. Plus, exercise is more pleasant when you ease into it than when you take off like a Japanese bullet train. At the end of your workout, allow at least 5 minutes to cool down gradually. If you abruptly stop exercising, you may feel dizzy or nauseated, and you could even faint.

How Little Exercise Can You Get Away With?

How many days a week should you exercise when you travel? The answer depends, of course, on how often you travel and how long you're gone. If you work out regularly at home and take an occasional trip, you can better afford to skip workouts on the road than if travel consumes half your life. Still, a good rule of thumb is to do 30 minutes of cardio exercise daily. Once you fall out of the habit of exercise, it's tough to regain your momentum.

However, you don't have to fit your 30 minutes into a single session.

Even three 10-minute workouts — climbing your hotel stairs after breakfast, power-walking around the airport — will suffice. In fact, if you don't already exercise regularly, 10-minute bursts of exercise can actually improve both your health and fitness. This was shown in a University of Virginia study dubbed "Spark 2000" because participants were instructed to perform fifteen 10-minute "sparks" of exercise each week: 7 to 10 cardio sessions, 2 to 4 strength training sessions, and 2 to 4 stretching sessions. In just three weeks, the forty subjects — mostly overweight women — improved their cardiovascular fitness 10 to 15 percent. Their total cholesterol levels dropped, on average, 15 points, translating to a reduced risk of heart disease by 20 percent. (For details about this study, read *The Spark*, by Glenn Gaesser and Karla Dougherty, 2001.)

Of course, if you're training for competition or have more ambitious fitness goals, you'll need to get in some longer workouts. Rather than squeeze several mini workouts into your day, you may have to wake up early and devote a longer block of time to exercise.

But here's some encouraging information for travelers: the length of your workouts isn't as important as the intensity. Research suggests that you can cut drastically the length of your workouts and retain your fitness for several months. In one study, subjects trained 40 minutes a day, 6 days a week, for 10 weeks, alternating running and bicycling at high intensities. Then, for the next 15 weeks, they cut back to either 26 minutes or 13 minutes while maintaining their intensity. When asked to run at nearly an all-out effort, they lasted just as long (4 to 8 minutes) as they had before slashing their training. Not surprisingly, the 13-minute group did lose endurance, lasting an average of 123 minutes at a moderate intensity, compared to 139 minutes for the other group. Still, considering they had cut the length of their workouts by 66 percent, a 10-percent drop in performance is pretty impressive. Meanwhile, the 26-minute group, having cut the length of their workouts by 33 percent, lost nothing.

Although they cut the length of their workouts, the subjects in this study were still exercising six days a week. If that's not realistic for your

> **But here's some encouraging information for travelers: the length of your workouts isn't as important as the intensity.**

travel schedule, reduce the number of days you exercise but keep the length of your workouts — and your intensity — the same. Research suggests that you can maintain most of your fitness, or at least a couple of months, on just two weekly workouts.

The bottom line: If you're tempted to blow off exercise on the road, these numbers should make you think twice. Remind yourself how little time it takes to maintain the fruits of your labor — and how frustrated you'll be if you let all your hard work go to waste.

How Hard Should You Push Yourself?

So, if intensity is the critical component in maintaining cardio fitness, just how much effort should you exert? Again, the answer depends on your goals. If you're aiming for general fitness, simply take the talk test: Push hard enough that you're slightly winded but not so breathless that you can't string together a complete sentence. If you're able to belt out Broadway show tunes, you'd better pick up the pace.

You may also want to try interval training, a particularly good strategy for time-pressed travelers. Whether you're on a bike, in a pool, or on a treadmill, alternate short, intense bursts of exercise — the kind that leave you gasping for breath — with segments of easier exercise. For instance, after your warm-up, push hard for 15 to 30 seconds and then ease up for 60 to 90 seconds. Or, do a less precise version of interval training using elements in your surroundings. If, say, you're jogging in Beverly Hills, sprint to every other lamppost, palm tree, or parked Lexus. You can gain more cardiovascular fitness and burn more calories if you do intervals than if you always exercise at the same pace. Just don't overdo it; even top athletes don't do hard interval training more than once or twice a week. Your body needs time to recover from intense exercise.

If the talk test strikes you as too vague, try gauging your intensity on a scale from 1 to 10. Assign a "1" to an activity that you could sustain for hours, like reclining on a lounge chair at Club Med. A "10" would involve major suffering, like sprinting up the steep and curvy Lombard Street in San Francisco, which contains ten hairpin turns in one block. Most of your workouts should rate between a 5 and an 8. Beginners should aim for the lower end of this range. If you're fairly fit, vary your workouts so that you sometimes reach the higher end. Before you travel, practice paying attention to how your body feels at different intensity levels. This way, when you're on your trip, you can easily replicate your usual intensity and better maintain your fitness.

If you're more serious about gauging your intensity, you may even want to invest in a heart-rate monitor, a device that straps around your chest and measures how fast your heart is beating. The number of beats per minute appears on a watch-size receiver you wear on your wrist. Aim to keep this number within your "target zone," a range of 50 to 80 percent of your maximum heart rate, the fastest your heart can possibly beat. The most popular formula for estimating your "max" is to subtract your age from 220. If you're 40 years old, your max is thought to be about 180, and the appropriate range for exercise would be 90 beats per minute (50 percent of your max) to 144 (80 percent). You could go as high as 90 percent — 162 beats per minute — during short intervals.

However, this time-honored formula is very rough — and for some people, wildly inaccurate. It was based on studies that included smokers and people with heart disease and was never intended to be used by the general public as a way to gauge appropriate intensity levels for a fitness program. Although experts say that no formula will be accurate for everyone, some put more stock in a newer calculation: Multiply your age by 0.7, and subtract this number from 208. The two formulas give basically the same numbers until age 40, above which the newer formula results in a higher estimated max.

The best way to determine your true max is to have a physician test you on a treadmill or an exercise bike, whichever you're most accustomed to using. The test takes 12 to 15 minutes, during which you increase your intensity every 30 to 60 seconds until you reach your max.

Heart-rate monitors are popular among competitive athletes; many divide their target zone into five mini zones and follow training programs that involve working in all of the zones. (For details about heart rate–based training, consult books written by Ed Burke, Sally Edwards, or Joe Friel.) However, many recreational exercisers also find heart-rate monitors helpful, especially when they travel.

Consider Chuck Hull, who spends nine months a year on the road as the tour manager for various rock bands and always travels with his bicycle. Hull says his workout schedule can be so erratic that he loses the ability to gauge his intensity accurately on a 1-to-10 scale. "When you've been off the bike for a week and you're in strange territory, sometimes you think you're pushing harder than you really are," Hull says. His heart-rate monitor gives him a reality check. Other times, he says, he's so excited to be back in the saddle that he starts off way too fast. "I look down at my monitor and realize I'm already pushing eighty-five percent of my max, so I back off."

Choosing Your Cardio Machine

What's the best cardiovascular equipment? For a traveler, the answer often depends on what's available. If the only cardio machine in your hotel is a rickety old bike, you may be more comfortable or motivated walking outside or climbing your hotel steps. If you have access to high-quality equipment, simply choose the machine that you enjoy most or that best suits your needs. The number of calories you burn depends more on how hard you push than on the specific machine you use.

A bike or stairclimber is ideal if you're using your cardio time for reading, whether you're preparing for a meeting or scanning a travel guide for sightseeing ideas. Some people have mastered the art of reading while walking on the treadmill. However, reading is not a swift idea if you're running,

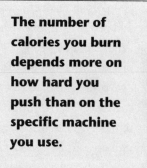

The number of calories you burn depends more on how hard you push than on the specific machine you use.

as staying upright on a treadmill can require some focus. Chris Lehane, Al Gore's press secretary during the 2000 presidential campaign, was once catapulted off a hotel treadmill in New Hampshire while watching TV. "It was right before the New Hampshire primary, and I was watching Bill Bradley do an interview on TV," Lehane recalls. "He made a really big mistake, and I got so excited that I lost my footing and the machine threw me right off."

Before you leave on a trip, familiarize yourself with the most popular cardio machines: treadmills, stairclimbers, stationary bikes, and elliptical trainers. Your hotel may have one of each, but if the stairclimber is the only one unoccupied and your time is short, you'll have to use it, whether or not it's your favorite. You'll be less likely to blow off your workout if you're comfortable on all of these contraptions.

How Many Calories Are You Burning?

How many minutes of exercise will it take to burn off all those Double Whoppers you inhaled on your cross-country road trip? A Double Whopper contains 920 calories, so, as the table below indicates, you have an awful lot of walking, swimming, or stairclimbing to do.

Of course, you can't use cardio exercise to compensate for lousy eating habits; you can end up with clogged arteries no matter how much time you spend on the treadmill. But knowing how many — or how few

Estimated Calories Burned		
1 min. 130 lbs / 180 lbs	15 mins. 130 lbs / 180 lbs	30 mins. 130 lbs / 180 lbs
Climbing stairs (30 steps/minute		
on 8-inch steps) 7.1 / 9.9	107 / 149	214 / 298
Jogging		
5 mph (12-min. mi.) 7.9 / 10.9	119 / 164	238 / 328
6 mph (10-min. mi.) 9.5 / 13.1	143 / 197	286 / 394
7 mph (8:35-min. mi.) 11 / 15.4	165 / 231	330 / 462
8 mph (7:30-min. mi.) 12.6 / 17.6	222 / 264	444 / 328
9 mph (6:40-min. mi.) 14 / 19.5	210 / 293	420 / 586
Jumping Rope 7.8 / 10.8	117 / 234	162 / 324
Swimming		
Freestyle, 35 yds./min. 6.4 / 8.8	96 / 132	192 / 264
Freestyle, 50 yds./min. 9.2 / 12.8	138 / 192	276 / 384
Breaststroke, 30 yds./min. 6.2 / 8.6	93 / 129	186 / 258
Breaststroke, 40 yds./min. 8.3 / 11.5	125 / 173	250 / 346
Walking		
3 mph (20-min. mi.) 3.5 / 4.9	53 / 74	106 / 148
3.2 mph (18:45-min. mi.) 4.1 / 5.6	62 / 84	124 / 168
3.5 mph (17:10-min. mi.) 4.4 / 6.2	66 / 93	132 / 186
4.0 mph (15-min. mi.) 5.5 / 7.6	83 / 114	166 / 228
4.5 mph (13:20-min. mi.) 6.2 / 8.6	93 / 129	186 / 258
5 mph (12-min mi.) 7.1 / 9.8	107 / 147	214 / 294

— calories you burn during a workout may give you incentive to keep exercising and improving your eating habits on the road.

Most cardio machines have a calorie-burning readout, so this table includes only activities that don't involve equipment. Keep in mind that the numbers — like those provided by cardio machines — are rough estimates. The number of calories you actually burn depends on many factors, including your weight, intensity level, fitness level, metabolism, muscle mass, and skill with the type of exercise you're performing. Some heart-rate monitors give calorie-burning estimates for whatever activity you happen to be doing; the most accurate versions are those that ask your age and weight.

Adapting Your Workouts to the Weather

When you're on the road, it's important to adjust your workouts according to internal factors, such as how tired or jet-lagged you feel. But you also need to consider external factors, such as changes in climate and altitude. Whether you've landed in steamy New Orleans or traveled to cold and dry Lake Tahoe, heeding the following advice will keep you comfortable while you exercise and minimize any climate-related risks to your health.

Handling Heat and Humidity

Working out in blistering weather can quickly leave you dehydrated and overheated. Here's how to protect yourself from the very serious dangers of heat.

Guzzle water. You sweat more in hot, humid climates, so compensate for the lost fluid by drinking extra water. If you're working out for more than 45 minutes, a sports drink is even better; you'll replenish electrolytes as well as fluids. Keep a water bottle with you at all times, and drink water before, during, and after your workouts. The jet lag section in Chapter 1 explains what happens to your body when you become dehydrated.

Go for shorter, easier workouts. Your body is working overtime to cool itself off, depleting your strength and stamina. Strenuous exercise under these conditions can lead to heat exhaustion. Symptoms include dizziness, nausea, weakness, muscle cramps, and irritability; if you experience any of these, lie down in the shade and drink cool water. Even more dangerous is heat stroke, a life-threatening condition triggered when your body's temperature-regulating mechanisms fail. You may experience difficulty breathing, extremely high body temperature, a rapid pulse, and hallucinations. Cool down immediately with water, a fan, air-conditioning, or ice packs, and get to the hospital.

Exercise in fabrics that wick away moisture. See Chapter 2 for examples of lightweight, synthetic fabrics that allow your sweat to evaporate quickly. Cotton can be uncomfortable in the heat because it absorbs sweat, becomes heavy, and sticks to your body.

Slather on sunblock. You don't want to spend your Hawaiian vacation inside your hotel room nursing blisters and sunburn (and worrying about having elevated your skin cancer risk). Sunblocks designed for exercise aren't totally sweatproof, so reapply the lotion often. Wear a hat and sunglasses, too.

Work out in the morning or evening. Avoiding midday workouts will reduce your risk of both heat-related illnesses and sunburn.

Cold-Weather Workouts

Unless your travels take you to Mount Everest or you happen to drop your gloves in a Porta Potti while on a ski trip, you're not likely to experience the most serious dangers of exercising in cold weather: frostbite and hypothermia. Still, being unprepared for the cold can make your workouts mighty unpleasant, even a bit hazardous.

Dress in layers. Even in freezing temperatures, you can work up quite a sweat while walking, jogging, skiing, or snowshoeing. If the layer touching your body gets soaked, you'll feel miserably cold, so start with a synthetic wicking fabric. The second layer serves as an insulator, trapping warm air generated by your body heat. A fleece vest or pullover works well, providing warmth and, depending on the design, wind protection, without too much bulk. You may also want to wear, or carry, a breathable jacket with underarm vents.

Your legs tend to warm up quickly, so thermal underwear and tights should suffice; you may not even need the thermals. A hat (or headband) and gloves are crucial; for both, you may find fleece softer than wool. To keep your toes toasty, go with Smartwool socks, made from a wool-synthetic blend that's designed for exercise and, unlike 100-percent wool, doesn't lose its shape.

Dressing properly is particularly important when the weather is both cold and damp. If you're not prepared, you can experience hypothermia when temperatures are in the forties and fifties.

Remember to drink water. You don't notice yourself sweating when you're clothed from head to toe, but rest assured, your body is perspiring and you risk dehydration if you don't drink enough. Cold, dry air doesn't hold as much water as warmer air, so when you breathe your body extracts water from your tissues to warm and humidify the air before it gets to your lungs. The result: a fluid deficit that can profoundly affect your stamina and judgment. It's not uncommon for ski patrollers to rescue dehydrated crash victims from the mountains. Carry a water bottle in your waist pack; better yet, wear an insulated, winter version of the hydration packs described in Chapter 2.

Shorten your workout. If you're walking in snow, you expend extra energy simply to keep yourself upright. On unplowed streets, your glutes and thigh muscles will work harder than usual, so you may poop out sooner than you expect.

Wear sunblock. The sun reflecting off the snow can leave you with a particularly painful burn.

Exercising at Altitude

The effects of altitude aren't as obvious as the effects of heat, humidity, and cold weather. Nevertheless, the potential hazards — dehydration and altitude sickness — are significant.

The air at elevation contains less oxygen than the air at sea level. Altitude sickness, also called acute mountain sickness, is your body's response to this oxygen deficit. The symptoms — headache, nausea, shortness of breath, drowsiness, confusion, slowed reflexes, decreased appetite — tend to kick in at elevations above 8,000 feet, but some people feel ill at altitudes as low as 5,000 feet. There's no telling who will get sick and who won't; being in shape doesn't make you immune. But one thing is for sure: Exerting yourself at altitude can exacerbate the symptoms. Here's how to exercise safely at high elevations.

Drink more water than usual. Inhaling dry air dries out your lungs. As in the cold, your body compensates by extracting fluid from your tissues, leaving you more susceptible to dehydration. Exercising in air that's both dry and cold makes the situation worse. Drink enough water so that your urine is nearly colorless.

Don't push so hard. It's more difficult to breathe in air that has less oxygen, so don't place excess demands on your body with intense exercise. You need at least three days — perhaps as many as seven — to adjust to the altitude before you can comfortably increase your intensity. The higher the elevation, the longer it takes your body to acclimate. Complete acclimatization typically takes a month. Even if you're free from mountain-sickness symptoms, don't expect to run or swim at the same pace you can maintain at sea level. The body simply cannot perform as well at altitude.

Be sure to eat enough. On the road, you're usually trying to stop yourself from overindulging, but you may find the opposite problem at high elevations. Altitude can decrease your appetite, but it doesn't decrease your body's need for fuel to exercise. If you don't consume enough calories, you'll fatigue during your workout.

6

Back to P.E.:
Jumping Rope, Climbing Stairs,
and Good Ol' Calisthenics

Let's consider the worst-case scenario on the cardio front. Your hotel has nothing but a cheapo bike with a broken seat — or no equipment at all. You can't go jogging because it's dark or the neighborhood is iffy. Or maybe you're in, say, Xi'an, China, where the sidewalks are cracking, the pollution is world-class, and the maniac drivers hop sidewalk curbs, speed down the wrong side of the road, and generally behave as if red lights are nothing but street decorations.

How can you possibly get in a workout? Actually, you still have several options. This chapter covers the best ones — jumping rope, climbing stairs, and stepping — along with a last-resort alternative that will take you back to elementary school P.E., only without the earsplitting screech of Mr. Duberstein's whistle.

Jumping Rope: The Killer Cardio Workout

A jump rope takes up less space in your luggage than a shaving kit and doesn't require much room to use — just enough to clear the rope overhead and in front of and behind you. This may require shoving aside furniture in your hotel room or taking your rope outside. Just be prepared for some curious stares if you jump in public. "Once I was staying at a really ratty hotel alongside a highway in the middle of an industrial area," says CC Cunningham, the Evanston, Illinois, trainer who designed the workouts in this chapter. "I was afraid of getting lost if I went running, so I jumped rope in the back parking lot. The truckers would pull in on their way to the warehouse, and they'd slow way, way down as they drove by."

Don't underestimate the challenge of jumping rope. Even if you are the star of your Spinning class or have endless stamina on the stair-climber, jumping rope may leave you breathless after a minute or two, and your calf muscles may be so sore the next day that you can barely walk. Before your trip, give yourself a few weeks to develop your rope jumping tolerance in small increments. You also need time to master the different footwork patterns; jumping rope is a skill that needs to be learned before it can be used as exercise. Don't count on your rope for an entire workout right away. Jumping rope is hard on your lower back, hips, knees, ankles, and feet and can lead to overuse injuries if you do too much too soon. For details on choosing the right rope, see Chapter 2.

Where to Jump

Jumping rope is most enjoyable on a smooth, shock-absorbent surface such as rubberized flooring and hardwood, but padded carpet will suffice. Dirt, gravel, or wood chips also work. Grass tends to catch the rope but is otherwise okay. Try to avoid jumping on asphalt or concrete, which is hard on your legs and feet.

What to Wear

Cross-training shoes are your best bet. Running shoes aren't ideal because they tend to have poor shock absorption in the forefoot area, where you land after each jump. If you feel pain in your lower leg, foot, or knee, try shoes with a wider and more cushioned forefoot. Don't jump rope barefoot; your feet need the support of athletic shoes.

Jump Rope Technique

Arm position: Keep your arms relaxed by your sides, your elbows bent, and your hands away from your body. Tensing your shoulders will raise the rope and may cause it to catch your feet. Turn the rope from your wrists, not your arms, and keep your arm movements small.

Leg position: Shift your weight onto the balls of your feet, soften your knees as you jump, and land with your knees slightly bent and heels slightly off the ground. Land lightly, not with a thud. The louder the noise, the more force you send up through your body.

Building Up Your Jumping Tolerance

Start with jumping sessions of 1 or 2 minutes, either at the end of your usual cardio workout at home or as intervals during a strength workout. As you gain fitness and proficiency with the footwork, gradually make the sessions longer, aiming for 5 minutes. To keep your heart rate up while you take a break between jumping stints, do rope swings (described in the next section).

While you develop your tolerance, watch for signs of an injury brewing. Sore feet, shins, knees, or hips could mean you're overdoing it. Also, check your footwear and surface. Once you have developed stamina for jumping rope, a 20-minute session will satisfy any workout craving.

Jump Rope Footwork

Like aerobic dance moves, jump rope patterns range from simple to complicated. The more jumps you learn, the better you can avoid boredom and repetitive stress on your legs. Try each of the following footwork patterns, giving yourself room to make mistakes. Eventually you'll be able to jump for several minutes, deftly changing from one pattern to another.

Rope Swings: Holding the handles together in both hands, swing the rope from side to side, bouncing slightly on your feet as you swing or step from side to side. Use rope swings for your warm-up or rest breaks.

Two-Foot Jump: Take off and land on both feet simultaneously.

Alternate-Foot Step: As you jump, alternate landing on your right foot and then your left, as if you're jogging.

Two Right, Two Left: Alternate two consecutive single-leg jumps on your right foot and two jumps on your left.

Skier's Jump: Jump side to side on both feet.

Forward Backward: Jump a few inches forward and then a few inches back on both feet.

V Jump: With both feet, jump diagonally forward to the left, then back to center, then diagonally forward to the right, then back to center.

Jump Rope Workouts

Preworkout Briefing

Here are three workouts to suit various time schedules and fitness levels. If you don't like any particular footwork pattern, substitute another. As you become comfortable with the various jumps, use them to create your own routines. After each workout, thoroughly stretch your hamstrings, quadriceps, shoulders, and calf muscles, following the flexibility exercises in Chapter 13. If you have time, stretch after your warm-up, before your main jumping set.

Just a Quickie: Try this one when you have just 10 to 15 minutes.

Warm-up: 50 Rope Swings

30 jumps each:
- Alternate-Foot Step
- Two-Foot Jump
- Two Right, Two Left
- Skier's Jump

50 jumps each:
- Alternate-Foot Step
- Two-Foot Jump
- Two Right, Two Left
- Skier's Jump

30 jumps each:
- Forward Backward
- V Jump
- Skier's Jump

20 jumps each, followed by 30 Rope Swings:
- Alternate-Foot Step
- Two-Foot Jump
- Two Right, Two Left
- Skier's Jump

50 jumps each:
- Forward Backward
- V Jump

100 jumps:
- Alternate-Foot Step or Two-Foot Jump

Cool-down: 50 Rope Swings

Goin', Goin', Goin': Repeat this 5-minute workout as many times as you can and see how long you can last.

Warm-up: 50 Rope Swings

80–100 jumps each:
- Alternate-Foot Step
- Two-Foot Jump
- Two Right, Two Left
- Skier's Jump

Recovery: 50 Rope Swings

80–100 jumps each:
- Forward Backward
- V Jump
- Alternate-Foot Step
- Two-Foot Jump

Repeat the workout as many times as you want.

Cool-down: 50 Rope Swings

Triple Whammy: This routine combines cardio exercise with stretching and strength training. Choose a couple of footwork patterns that are easy for you to do. For the strength work, do the tubing exercises in Chapter 11 or the hotel-room exercises in Chapter 12. This workout should take 30 to 45 minutes, depending on the number of strength exercises and sets you perform.

Warm-up: For 3 minutes, alternate 50 Rope Swings with 100 jumps using easy footwork patterns.
Do all of the stretches in Chapter 13.
Do 100 jumps between every one or two strength exercises.

Breaking a Sweat on Stairs and Steps

If jumping rope doesn't suit you or you don't have a rope, you can get a plenty tough cardio workout on the stairs in your hotel or motel. This section covers two types of stair workouts: stair climbing and stepping. Stair-climbing workouts involve one or more flights of multiple steps. Step workouts involve a single step or steplike object, such as a step aerobics platform, which you may be able to find in larger hotel gyms. After each of these workouts, do all of the lower-body stretches in Chapter 13.

Climbing Stairs

Climbing flights of stairs is one of the hardest workouts around — tougher than stair-climbing machines because you have to lift your body weight up the steps. (On most machines, your feet stay glued to the pedals.) Plus, you can't cheat by lean-ing on the console. Los Angeles bike racer Annelie Chapman ran the stairs daily in the Moscow apartment building where she spent six weeks while researching her doctoral disser-tation. Chapman, who rides her bike about three hours a day at home, says stair climbing, combined with 20 minutes of jumping rope, was a great way to work her cycling muscles and maintain adequate fitness during her cycling hiatus. However, she did attract some unwanted attention. One day she reached the last flight of stairs panting, only to be greeted by the overseer of the building, who demanded an explanation. "She let me go," Chapman says. "But she had

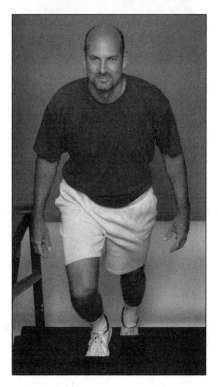

a skeptical look on her face, and I later found out she interrogated my host about me."

Preworkout Briefing

While stairs can be more challenging than stair-climbing machines, they also can pose more dangers. Most falls occur while walking down stairs because it's easy to lose your balance. A good stair-climbing work-out will maximize ascending and minimize descending. Here are some other tips for safe climbing.

- Choose a well-lit stairwell that allows you to exit on any floor. (In big cities, an isolated stairwell may pose safety concerns, so check with the hotel management before you work out.)

- Wear clothing that breathes, as you'll be working up a major sweat.

- Bring plenty of water, especially since there's little ventilation in a stairwell. You'll last longer if you're well hydrated. Instead of carrying your water bottle (it's best to keep your hands free in case you trip), keep the bottle at the top of the staircase.

- To increase the intensity of your workout, wear a lightly loaded backpack. For comfort and balance, place the heaviest item toward the top of the pack.

- When ascending, place your foot firmly on the center of the step, not on the edge. You may want to brush the railing with your hand as you ascend, but don't use it to propel yourself up the steps.

- When descending, grasp the handrail for balance. To give your thighs a rest, you may also want to try side-stepping down.

Stair-Climbing Workouts

High Rise: If your hotel has multiple floors and an elevator, take the stairs up and the elevator down. The effort going up will be enough to warrant the rest break on the way down; plus, you avoid the hazards of descending. Warm up by walking an easy three to five floors, then tackle as many flights as you can before heading down the elevator and climbing up again. Walking up stairs is plenty tough for most people, but if you're really fit, you may want to run up some or all of the flights. For variety, alternate between walking and running up each flight. Or, walk two flights and run one.

Low Rise: If you have five floors or fewer, this workout may be your best bet. Use flights instead of floors: Go up two flights and down one. Then go up two more and down another. Repeat until you have climbed all the way up. Then come down by elevator or side-step to give your legs a break. If there is a second stairwell at the opposite end of the hallway, climb up one floor, jog down the hall, and walk or run up the stairs at the opposite end. When you have reached the top, carefully descend to the bottom and begin again.

One Floor Up: If you're stuck with only one floor, make the best of it by repeatedly walking or jogging up and down. For variety, use side-stepping on both the up and down phases.

Step Workouts

A step workout requires more creativity than stair climbing, but if you don't have access to a staircase, it can be a decent way to get sweaty. You also can alternate stepping with jumping rope, especially if you're a beginner with the rope and have limited endurance.

You may have to be creative with finding your step. A step can be any object that is stable, with a sturdy top, and can support at least 1.5 times your bodyweight. A step shouldn't be more than 12 inches high. At some high-end hotels, you can even request that a step aerobics platform be delivered to your room, along with a video.

Preworkout Briefing

Follow these tips for safe and effective stepping.

- When stepping up, place your foot firmly on the step, not on the edge.

- Stay toward the center of the step, away from the ends.

- Switch your lead foot (the one that steps up first) frequently.

- Swing, pump, or punch your arms as you step to increase the intensity of the workout. But don't bother packing hand weights, which offer a negligible calorie-burning benefit and can place undue stress on delicate joints such as your shoulder and elbow.

Putting Together Your Step Routine

Use the following steps to create your workouts. Most of them you can do on the bottom step of a flight of stairs, although a couple require a platform that you can step over.

Front
- Up, up, down, down
- Up, tap, down, tap
- Up, lift opposite leg, down tap

Sideways
- Up, tap, down, tap (stay on one side of the step)
- Up, up, down, down (start straddling the step)
- Up, lift, down, tap (stay on one side of the step)
- Up, up, down, tap on top of the step (traveling across the step from one side to the other)

Back to P.E.

Sometimes you're left with no other choice than to resort to the ways of the past. We're talking about jumping jacks, mountain climbers, and other oldies from P.E. Repeat the following workout sequence as long as you like. If possible, add a hallway jog to the circuit. Or, between calisthenics, insert one or two of the strength exercises in Chapters 11 or 12.

- **Low-Jump Twists (20 to each side):** With your feet together and knees slightly bent, hop slightly and rotate your feet in one direction. On the next hop, rotate in the opposite direction. Keep your shoulders still as you rotate. Do 20 to each side.

- **Jumping Jacks (20)**

- **Wall Jogs (1 minute):** Stand about two feet from a wall and lean forward, placing your hands against the wall at shoulder height. Jog in place while you "push" against the wall. The higher you lift your knees, the tougher the workout.

- **Mountain Climbers (25 with each foot):** Place your hands on the floor or the edge of a desk or dresser. Start with your right foot staggered in front of your left. Jump up and switch feet, bringing your left leg forward. Repeat, alternating feet.

- **Side Shuffles (10):** Using as much space as you have available, shuffle to the side, keeping your feet apart. Then reverse directions. Go side-to-side repeatedly.

7

Swimming Laps — and What to Do When the Pool Is Too Small

As a stand-up comic, Laurie Kilmartin has spent up to forty weeks a year on the road, entertaining audiences from Boise to Baton Rouge to Bahrain. But there has been one constant in her topsy-turvy schedule: swimming. "Nothing takes the sting out of homesickness like losing yourself in a swim workout," says Kilmartin, who lives in New York City. That black line at the bottom of the pool, she says, looks the same everywhere. "Swimming on the road has saved me thousands of dollars on therapy and pharmaceuticals, and not in that order. Whenever I land, my second phone call is to the local YMCA. Of course, my first is to my agent and usually starts with 'Al, why am I working this dump?'"

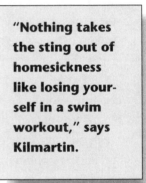

"Nothing takes the sting out of homesickness like losing yourself in a swim workout," says Kilmartin.

But seriously, folks . . . Swimming can be an ideal travel workout — a soothing way to recover from a difficult journey, an opportunity to mull over a presentation without being interrupted by your cell phone or pager. Your swimsuit and goggles consume minimal space in your suitcase. Plus, in a pool, you can't get lost.

Still, for many exercisers, swimming seems to have one huge drawback: It's so darned boring. The black line that keeps Kilmartin from getting homesick can lull some people practically into a coma. Yet swimming doesn't have to seem like forced labor. Instead of slogging through lap after lap after mind-numbing lap, you can break your routine into faster-paced mini workouts, each with its own focus. This approach saves you precious time, improves your fitness, and makes swimming more enjoyable.

This chapter teaches you to design swimming workouts that fit into any travel schedule. Like weight routines in the gym, swim workouts have a basic structure. You simply adjust the variables — the pace, rest periods, distances, and strokes. You also can spice up your workouts with gadgets such as a kickboard and pull buoy, a small float that you stick between your legs to keep them still while you focus on your upper body. Most full-size pools have these toys available. If you're using a hotel pool, pack the nifty inflatable versions shown in Chapter 2. The workouts in this chapter were designed by Kerry O'Brien, coach of the Walnut Creek Master's swim club in northern California.

Of course, lap swimming isn't always realistic for travelers. You may not have the time or transportation to get to a local pool, or the pool may be so crowded that you'd have to mow down a half dozen hotel guests to complete a lap. In addition, some hotel pools are so small that you can traverse the length in six strokes.

For these situations, we suggest aquatic exercise. No, aquatic exercise is not something performed by ninety-year-olds in shower caps. It's a catchall term for cardiovascular and muscle-conditioning moves you can do in chest-high water — and send your heart rate soaring in the process. "If you've got a five-foot-by-five-foot area of water, you can get a great workout," says Angie Proctor,

> "If you've got a five-foot-by-five-foot area of water, you can get a great workout," says Angie Proctor, executive director of the Aquatic Exercise Association.

executive director of the Aquatic Exercise Association. Proctor, who designed the aquatic routines in this chapter, has exercised in bodies of water that don't even deserve to be called swimming pools. "At one hotel in New Orleans I paid three hundred bucks a night, and the pool was barely bigger than a Jacuzzi," says Proctor, who travels five months a year. "But I still got in my workout." With Proctor's challenging routine, you'll be able to do the same.

Anatomy of a Swim Workout

Swim workouts typically are divided into sets, separated by rest periods of a few minutes. There's no law dictating how many sets a swim workout should include; serious swimmers typically do five or six sets of varying lengths. Below is a simplified, three-set format that may be more practical for busy travelers. You can use this format regardless of your fitness level or time constraints. However, if you have plenty of time or are a fit swimmer, you may want to check out the U.S. Masters Swimming Web site, usms.org. In the training section, you'll find dozens of sample workouts of varying lengths, along with links to other training sites. Even if you're a novice swimmer, you can use the Masters workouts to give you ideas for creating your own routines.

Typically, swim workouts are noted in yards rather than laps. For instance, a swim coach will say, "Do a five-hundred warm-up," meaning "warm up by swimming 500 yards," which — in the standard 25-yard pool — is 20 laps. However, because the pools that travelers encounter (particularly hotel pools) may vary greatly in length, the workouts in this chapter are denoted in laps. One lap equals one length of the pool. Here's a look at the three-set format:

Warm-up Set (10 to 20 percent of total yardage): Swim at an easy pace, getting a feel for the water. Include all of the strokes you plan to use in your workout. You also can include kicking (with a kickboard) and/or pulling (with a pull buoy between your legs). Here are some sample warm-ups:

- Swim 8 laps at an easy pace
- Swim 4 laps, kick 4 laps
- Swim 8 laps, alternating 1 lap freestyle with 1 lap backstroke or breaststroke

Main Set (60 to 75 percent of total yardage): This set is the longest, most intense part of your workout. Choose a focus, such as speed work, endurance training, or particular strokes.

While you generally swim continuously during your warm-up (and cool-down), your main set is typically broken into intervals, with short rests between them. Here are some sample main sets based on specific daily goals.

- **Speed:** Swim 16 laps broken into 8 intense, 2-lap intervals, resting 15 seconds between intervals. Or swim the first lap of each interval all-out, then swim at an easy pace on the return, resting 10 seconds until you take off again.
- **Endurance:** Swim 24 laps in 3 intervals of 8 laps each at a moderate pace, resting 1 minute between intervals. Or swim 2 intervals of 10 laps each, aiming to swim the second one faster than the first.
- **Stroke work:** Do 6 intervals of 3 laps (1 lap backstroke, 1 lap breaststroke, 1 lap freestyle), resting 20 seconds between intervals. Or do 8 intervals of 2 laps, alternating 2 laps of easy freestyle swimming with 2 moderate-to-hard laps of backstroke or breaststroke, resting 15 seconds between intervals.

Cool-down Set (10 percent of total yardage): This short, slow set is your victory lap, your pat on the back. A typical cool-down is 4 yards of easy freestyle swimming.

Preworkout Briefing

Before you get in the pool, loosen up for a few minutes by gently rotating both arms, going forward and backward. Then cross your arms in front of you and behind you several times.

The Pyramid Workout, the Multispeed Workout, and the Mixed-Stroke Workout follow the three-set format. If you're swimming in a 25-yard pool, a 50-lap workout (1,200 yards) should take about 30 minutes. Rest a few minutes between sets. Be sure to wear a watch so that you can keep track of your rest periods. If you're swimming in a pool that's regularly used for lap swimming — such as a YMCA pool, health club, or university pool — you'll probably have access to a pace clock, the large clock set up at the end of the pool.

"Kicking" means holding on to a kickboard and using only your legs. "Pulling" means placing a pull buoy between your legs and using only your arms. If you don't have access to this equipment, simply swim freestyle.

Pyramid Workout

The main set of this 46-lap (1,150-yard) endurance workout features a "pyramid": You gradually build up from 2 laps to 8 laps and then go back down to 2. To make the workout longer, take the pyramid to 10 laps instead of 8.

Warm-up (easy pace)

- 4 laps freestyle
- 4 laps kicking
- 2 laps pulling

Main set (moderate pace)

- 2 laps freestyle, rest 5 seconds
- 4 laps freestyle, rest 10 seconds
- 6 laps freestyle, rest 15 seconds
- 8 laps freestyle, rest 20 seconds
- 6 laps freestyle, rest 15 seconds
- 4 laps freestyle, rest 10 seconds
- 2 laps freestyle, rest 5 seconds

Cool-down (easy pace)

- 4 laps freestyle

Multispeed Workout

During this 52-lap (1,300-yard) freestyle workout you vary your intensity level.

Warm-up (easy pace)

- 4 laps freestyle
- 4 laps pulling
- 4 laps kicking

Main set

- 6 laps freestyle (easy pace), rest 10 seconds
- 4 laps freestyle (moderate pace), rest 20 seconds
- 2 laps freestyle (fast pace), rest 30 seconds
- Repeat all of the above a total of 3 times

Cool-down (easy pace)

- 4 laps freestyle

Mixed-Stroke Workout

This 36-lap (900-yard) workout includes freestyle, breaststroke, and backstroke. If you don't enjoy doing one of the strokes, substitute another.

Warm-up (easy pace)
- 4 laps, alternating freestyle and breaststroke
- 4 laps, alternating freestyle and backstroke

Main set
- 2 laps breaststroke (first lap moderate pace, second lap fast pace)
- 2 laps backstroke (first lap moderate pace, second lap fast pace)
- Rest 30 seconds
- Repeat all of the above a total of 6 times

Cool-down (easy pace)
- 4 laps freestyle

Swimming Technique Tips

Here are a few tips to make your freestyle swimming more effective.

- Focus on rolling your body side to side as you pull through the water. Don't just lie flat on the water while spinning your arms.

- Lengthen your stroke. Reach as far in front of you as possible, taking long, efficient strokes rather than short, choppy ones. Pull all the way through the water, brushing your thumb against your thigh to make sure you finish the stroke. Keep your head still as your body rotates from side to side.

- A few times during each workout, count the number of strokes you take per length. The fewer the better. Beginners typically take 21 to 24 strokes to get across a 25-yard pool. As you become more efficient, you may get your stroke count down to 18 or 19.

Aquatic Exercise: What to Do When the Pool Is Too Small for Swimming

If you don't enjoy lap swimming or are stuck with a hotel pool that's too small, try this timesaving workout, which combines aerobic exercise with muscle-conditioning moves. You can adjust the routine so that it lasts from 25 to 60 minutes. Equipment isn't necessary, although webbed gloves can help you maintain balance and boost the intensity of your workout. You can purchase these gloves for about $20 through hydrofit.com and hydrotone.com.

Preworkout Briefing

The ideal water depth for this workout is about midchest. If the water is too shallow, stick to the aerobics moves with the least amount of impact, such as the Pendulum or Skates (see the bulleted list that follows). For the muscle-conditioning segment, bend your hips and knees further so that the muscles and joints you are working are fully submerged. If the water is deeper than midchest level, slow down the moves to make sure you work through the full range of motion.

Perform the aerobic movements at a brisk pace, about 60 to 70 foot touches per minute. Working out to music will help you stay motivated. Try using a waterproof tape or CD player with music tempos of 125 to 140 beats per minute. You can buy CDs specially designed for aquaworkouts at dynamixmusic.com, which lists the tempo of each song.

Always warm up for at least 5 minutes using any of the moves listed under "Cardio Movement Choices." Then perform the Cardio and Muscle-Conditioning Workout. For the cardio segments, choose the moves you like best, performing 16 to 32 repetitions of one move before switching to another. For the muscle-conditioning segments, perform 30 repetitions of each exercise. Repeat the routine as time permits.

Cardio Movement Choices

Knee Lift: Jog in place while exaggerating your knee lift.

Knee Lift with Kick: Do three consecutive knee lifts and, on the fourth count, kick straight out.

Wide Jog: Jog in place with your legs wider than your hips. Lift your knees up to your hips.

Heel-back Jog: Jog in place, kicking your feet up to your butt.

Skates: Push back diagonally with one leg at a time, as if you're speedskating.

Pendulum: Swing your body from side to side, lifting your arms and legs in opposition. As you raise your left leg out to the side, raise your right arm, then switch sides.

Jazz Kick: Kick diagonally with alternating legs, as if you're doing the cancan.

Bounce Wide: With your legs comfortably wide, jump straight up off the bottom of the pool. Bend your knees as you land to soften the impact.

Bounce Close: With your legs directly under your hips, jump straight up, bending your knees as you land.

Cardio and Muscle-Conditioning Workout

- Cardio moves, 10 minutes
- Muscle-Conditioning Group A
- Cardio moves, 5 minutes
- Muscle-Conditioning Group B
- Cardio moves, 5 minutes
- Muscle-Conditioning Group C

Muscle-Conditioning Group A

Squat and Chest Press: Press your arms together at chest level while squatting, as if you're sitting in a chair, until your thighs are parallel to the pool bottom. When your shoulders hit the water surface, lift your arms out to the side and stand back up.

Plié and Press Down: Stand with your feet wider than your hips, toes pointing out, and arms straight out in front at shoulder level. As you press your arms down and back behind your body, lower into a plié until your hips are about 3 inches above your knees. Slowly return to the starting position.

Muscle-Conditioning Group B

Lunge and Lateral Raise: Stand with your arms hanging down at your sides and your feet hip-width apart with one foot a giant step in front of the other. Lower into a lunge position as you lift your arms out to the side to shoulder level. Make sure your front knee does not shoot over your toes. Return to the starting position.

Reverse Lunge and Front Raise: Stand with your feet together and arms hanging down. Step backward with one foot and lower into a lunge position as you lift both arms forward to shoulder level. Return to the starting position and switch legs, alternating as you complete the set.

Muscle-Conditioning Group C

Leg Lift and Biceps Curl: Stand with your feet hip-width apart and arms hanging down. Lift your left leg out to the side to just below hip height, keeping your toes facing forward at all times. As you lift your leg, bend your elbows, curling your hands toward your shoulders. Perform all repetitions with your left leg before switching legs. Then, instead of performing another set of biceps curls, do the Triceps Pushdown (see below) as you lift your right leg.

Leg Lift and Triceps Pushdown: Stand with your feet hip-width apart and arms bent, elbows pointing down and hands at your shoulders, palms facing forward. As you lift your right leg out to the side, press your arms down until they are straight. Keep your elbows glued to your sides throughout the motion.

More Cardio Moves

Here's a list of additional cardio movements you can add to your aquatic workout.

Jog: Run across the width of the pool, swinging your arms back and forth.

Sprint: Run across the pool forward and backward as fast as you can. Your knees won't lift as high and your arms won't swing as wide as when you jog at a slower pace.

Jumping Jack: To increase the intensity, travel across the pool as you do your jumping jacks.

Cross-Country Ski: Mimic the movement of a cross-country ski machine, exaggerating your arm movements.

Frog Jump: Jump off the pool bottom with your knees to the outside of your hips as you land.

Staying Strong on the Road

Cardiovascular exercise gives you the stamina for those marathon walks from the departure gate to baggage claim, but a healthy heart and lungs aren't particularly useful for hoisting heavy suitcases off the baggage-claim carousel. For that — and for plenty of other travel situations — you need strong muscles. Part III explains how to develop and maintain muscle strength on the road, whether you have access to top-notch gym equipment or nothing but the bed and desk in your hotel room.

Chapter 8 is a strength-training primer geared toward the traveler. It answers questions such as: How many days a week should you strength-train on the road? If you're pressed for time, which exercises should get top priority? Chapter 8 also covers important safety tips that apply to all methods of strength training. The next four chapters focus on specific types of equipment and include routines of varying lengths. Chapter 9 uncovers the mysteries of hotel multistation weight machines. Chapter 10 features dumbbell routines. Chapter 11 teaches you to use rubber exercise tubing, the most versatile strength-training method for travelers. Chapter 12 shows you how to make do without any equipment at all.

8

A Traveler's Strength-Training Guide

When the Lynyrd Skynyrd tour bus barrels down the highway en route to the next gig, most of the band members hang out in the rear of the bus watching satellite TV. But drummer Michael Cartellone can sometimes be found up front on the floor — cranking out pushups and abdominal crunches. "If we're on an all-day drive, I either have to do my workout on this two-and-a-half-foot-by-five-foot patch of carpet or miss a day," says Cartellone, thirty-eight. "Sometimes the bus is hitting bumps and I'm getting thrown side to side, but I have to do it."

For the firm and defined Cartellone, who usually performs shirtless, strength training has its obvious benefits. But muscle tone isn't what drives his daily workouts. Cartellone is counting on his routine to help prevent the tendinitis and arthritis that often afflict veteran drummers. "Drumming is the most physical activity you can do as a musician," he says. "The reason I can play with the stamina and power I do is because I'm in a constant training mode."

Even if your job isn't as physically demanding as Cartellone's — and involves performing your duties fully clothed — do your best to maintain a strength program on the road. Strength training is important for a long list of reasons, such as keeping your bones healthy, preserving your muscle mass and metabolism as you age, and mustering the oomph to screw off stubborn ketchup lids. When you're lugging suitcases through airport terminals and hoisting carry-on bags into overhead bins, you have even more reasons to challenge your muscles against resistance.

Any traveler needs a particularly good grasp of strength-training fundamentals. On the road you'll encounter unfamiliar equipment, and your schedule may be less predictable than it is at home. You need the skills to adapt your routine to any circumstance that comes up. Aim to get comfortable with a variety of strength-training tools, so you can piece together a solid workout with dumbbells, weight machines, rubber tubing, or just a patch of carpet on a rock-band tour bus.

> On the road you'll encounter unfamiliar equipment, and your schedule may be less predictable than it is at home.

This chapter covers the basics, so you can make the most of the exercises shown in Chapters 9 through 12. You'll learn how to distinguish high-priority exercises from the less crucial moves you can perform if you have the time. The safety advice in this chapter applies to all methods of strength training; the next four chapters include safety tips specific to the equipment discussed in them. One souvenir you definitely don't want to bring home is a strength-training injury.

Designing Your Strength Program

How many days a week do you really need to strength-train when you travel? How many different exercises should you do, and how many sets and repetitions of each? How much weight should you lift? The answers depend, of course, on your goals, your travel schedule, and your training program at home. You also need to consider how tired you are. If you've just set a world record for museums visited in a twelve-hour period, adapt your strength routine accordingly. (Just don't use your busy itinerary as an excuse to blow off your workouts altogether.) Use the guidelines below to tailor your program to your own needs. A trainer can help further personalize your routine.

Aim for two strength sessions a week. Even if you lift three times a week at home, twice a week is plenty when you're traveling. Research shows that beginners can get virtually the same benefit from training twice a week as they can from lifting three times. In fact, experienced lifters are better off hitting each muscle group twice a week so that their muscles have more time to recover from strenuous workouts. Even one weekly session on the road is better than nothing. In one study of experienced lifters, subjects who performed three sets of several exercises once a week achieved 62 percent of the strength gains reaped by subjects who performed one set of each exercise three days a week. Do fit in that one session, though. Otherwise, you'll be exceedingly sore after your first day back, and you'll waste a few sessions rebuilding your tolerance.

Do enough exercises to hit each of your major muscle groups. If you're pressed for time, choose moves that work several muscle groups at once. Most exercises that strengthen large muscle groups, such as your back, chest, and butt muscles, also work smaller muscles, such as your biceps, chest, shoulders, and thigh muscles. For instance, the pushup is primarily a chest exercise, but it also works your shoulders and triceps.

When you perform "multimuscle" exercises, your smaller muscles aren't as challenged as when you perform exercises that specifically target the small muscles; in other words, a triceps exercise strengthens your triceps better than a pushup does. However, when time is tight, something is better than nothing. Multimuscle exercises also deserve higher priority than single-muscle moves because they are more practical for getting through everyday life. When you lift a suitcase off the ground and shove it into the trunk of a taxi, just about all of your muscles come into play. It's not often in life that you use one muscle group at a time.

The multimuscle exercises in this book generally do not involve your abdominals in a significant way, so try to make time for exercises that focus on your abs. (See the Index of Exercises at the end of the book.) Isolating your abs is not the ideal way to strengthen them, but it's the simplest approach when you're on the road. When you're at home and have more time, try yoga, Pilates, or other disciplines that strengthen your core muscles — your abs, lower back, and butt muscles — in combination and more thoroughly.

Learn which exercises work which muscle groups so you can use your workout time wisely. Chapters 9 through 12 include mini workouts to help you prioritize when you're in a hurry.

Here are examples of exercises that save time because they work more than one muscle group.

Muscles Worked: Back, Biceps
- Lat Pulldown (Chapter 9)
- Seated Row Machine (Chapter 9)
- One-Arm Dumbbell Row (Chapter 10)
- Tubing Row (Chapter 11)

Muscles Worked: Chest, Shoulders, Triceps
- Seated Chest Press Machine (Chapter 9)
- Dumbbell Chest Press (Chapter 10)
- Pushup (Chapter 12)

Muscles Worked: Glutes, Quadriceps, Hamstrings
- Leg Press Machine (Chapter 9)
- Dumbbell Squat (Chapter 10)
- Dumbbell Lunge (Chapter 10)
- Tubing Squat (Chapter 11)
- Tubing Split Lunge (Chapter 11)
- Traveling Lunge (Chapter 12)
- Split Lunge (Chapter 12)

Muscles Worked: Lower Back, Glutes
- Alternating Back Extension (Chapter 12)
- Kneeling Back Extension (Chapter 12)

Do 1 to 3 sets per muscle group. If you're a beginning lifter or a veteran who's simply trying to maintain strength on a short trip, a single set will suffice. Do more sets if you have the time and enjoy a more elaborate routine. You may also want to beef up your program if traveling is your lifestyle rather than an interruption of your regular schedule. Research suggests that one set may be enough for beginners to make progress, but advanced lifters tend to plateau after a few months and generally need extra sets to continue gaining strength.

Rest 30 to 60 seconds between sets. Or, if you're really short on time, try circuit training, taking no rest at all between sets. Perform one set of an exercise, then move directly to a different exercise. Once you have completed the "circuit" — the whole routine — you may want to perform it a second or third time. Because you're not resting, you won't be able to lift as much weight with circuit training, but you'll save a lot of time. (Don't try to save time by speeding up your repetitions.)

Use enough resistance to fatigue your muscles at between 8 and 12 repetitions. Traveling isn't the time to set personal strength records. However, you won't stay strong and toned if you do repetitions with a dumbbell lighter than an airline-size bottle of Scotch. In fact, research suggests that to achieve the bone-strengthening benefits of strength-training, you need to be in the 8-repetition range regularly.

Strength-Training Safety Tips

You didn't travel halfway across the country — or the world — to lie flat on your back in your hotel room and watch the Weather Channel all day. Nothing can ruin a trip like a pulled muscle. To minimize your injury risk, heed the cautions below. Also, pay careful attention to the instructions for each exercise described in this book. You may want to hire a certified trainer for a couple of sessions to scrutinize your technique before you hit the road.

Always warm up. Before your strength-training workout, do at least 3 to 5 minutes of easy cardio exercise, even if it's the jumping jacks and other calisthenics in Chapter 6. Warmer muscles are more pliable and less susceptible to injury.

Do your repetitions slowly. When you zoom through your reps, you rely more on momentum than muscle power, and you increase your risk for making a wrong move. Take 2 seconds to perform an exercise and 2 to 4 seconds to return to the starting position. Taking an extra second or two to lower the weight can help you gain strength. On the lowering portion of an exercise, your muscles can handle about 40 percent more weight than they can on the lifting phase. Since you can't add 40 percent more weight in the middle of a repetition, the best way to make the lowering portion more challenging is to slow down.

Don't lift too much weight. Jet lag, sleep deprivation, and travel stress can zap your strength. Instead of mindlessly grabbing your usual weight, assess how you feel and drop down a few pounds if necessary. When you lift more weight than you can handle at the time, your technique gets sloppy. Also, you don't want to end up so sore the next day that you can barely shuffle across the hotel lobby.

Don't hold your breath. Lifting weights causes a momentary increase in your blood pressure, which normally is not a problem. But if you hold your breath as you lift, your blood pressure can skyrocket and then suddenly plunge, a scenario that may cause you to pass out. Breathe out when you strain to lift the weight, and inhale as you return the weight to the starting position.

A Traveler's Guide to the Major Muscle Groups

Sure, strength training gives you firm, toned muscles, but good looks will get you only so far on a business trip. This section explains how strong pecs, delts, and lats can make a difference when you travel.

Shoulders (deltoids or delts): You rely on your delts when you place luggage overhead and when you keep your arm up in the air while you try in vain to hail a cab.

Chest (pectorals or pecs): You need strong pecs for pushing motions, like shoving your luggage into place in the trunk of a car or pressing down on your overstuffed suitcase while your annoyed spouse tries to zip it shut.

Upper and middle back (trapezius or traps, latissimus dorsi or lats): You use your back muscles when you pull — for instance, when you open a heavy hotel door or hoist your suitcase onto the conveyor belt at baggage check-in. Strong traps also help prevent the achiness common after walking long distances with a laptop computer slung over your shoulder.

Biceps: Your biceps bend your elbow, so you need them for carrying that heavy stack of magazines for your 22-hour flight to Hong Kong. Your biceps also assist your back muscles when you yank on something stubborn, like the zipper on that overstuffed bag or a kid who'd rather play Nintendo in the car than visit the natural history museum.

Triceps: Your triceps straighten your elbow and assist your chest when you push something, like your overloaded luggage cart at baggage claim. Strong triceps also help prevent the elbow pain you can get from carrying a heavy briefcase while your arm is straight.

Lower back: Strong lower back muscles help you sit or stand with better posture and less back pain for extended periods. Your lower back muscles also work with your abdominals to keep your spine stable when you move the rest of your body, like when you reach around on the plane to tell the person behind you to stop kicking your seat.

Abdominals (abs): Your abs work with your lower back to support you during long periods of sitting and standing. They also help support all the weird contortions you go through to lift, carry, drag, toss, and grab your luggage.

Butt and hips (gluteals or glutes): You need strong glutes for climbing staircases and broken airport escalators and for walking up hills, such as the ramp of the airport parking lot. You also use your glutes when you squat down to pick up heavy bags and when you stand up to climb over your fellow airplane passengers en route to the bathroom.

Front thighs (quadriceps or quads): Strong quads are crucial on interminable walks to baggage claim and to famous shrines, especially if you get lost and all the signs are in Arabic. Strengthening your quads can help prevent the knee problems that may develop on your ski or hiking vacation.

Rear thighs (hamstrings): Your hamstrings assist in walking, climbing, and kicking the covers off your hotel bed when they've been tucked in too tight.

Calves: Strong calf muscles are important for long walks and for standing on your tiptoes to peer over the crowd and get a glimpse of breakdancing street performers. With powerful calves, you can spring off the ground in celebration when your delayed flight has been called for boarding.

9

Demystifying the
Hotel Multi-Gym

Over the course of your travels, you may encounter some daunting and mysterious sights, like Stonehenge or the giant statues on Easter Island or the world's first UFO landing pad in Alberta, Canada. However, few sights may be as puzzling as a hotel multistation weight machine, also known as a multi-gym. At first glance, you might think a fitness-crazed sculptor had turned a dozen health club machines upside down and sideways and welded them all together.

Confusing as they may seem, multi-gyms are popular in hotels because they are safer than dumbbells and barbells. They're also less expensive than a full line of weight machines, and they take up much less space because most of the bars and cables do double duty. For instance, you can work your upper back and your triceps with the same equipment simply by changing your body position. Although these machines are cleverly designed, it's not always obvious which way to sit or which handles to grasp for a particular exercise. This chapter takes the mystery out of these contraptions, giving you step-by-step instructions for the most common multi-gym exercises.

Be aware that not all multi-gyms are created equal. The more expensive brands tend to operate as smoothly as top health club machines. But some of the knockoffs generate a lot of friction, making the weight seem exceedingly heavy. Also, some models are sturdier and more solidly constructed than others. San Diego trainer Ken Baldwin was performing a one-handed biceps curl on a hotel multi-gym when the handle suddenly broke off from the cable. "The piece snapped while my arm was going up and I hit my chin," says Baldwin, who was, naturally, startled.

Low-end brands may also be engineered with less concern for your joints, so pay attention to how your body feels during each exercise. If a certain movement puts your knee in an awkward position or makes your shoulder feel as if it's going to be yanked out of its socket, skip the exercise and choose an alternative from Chapter 12. Be sure to adjust seats and handles so the machine fits your body. Finally, don't invent your own uses for any parts of the multi-gym. "I've seen people do some strange things," says Baldwin, who designed the workouts in this chapter. He watched one hotel guest stand on the chest-press bench, bend over, and pull up the handles to perform a makeshift back exercise. By creating your own exercises, you may inadvertently create back problems or cause other injuries.

The exercises in this chapter are among the most popular featured in multistation gyms. However, not every hotel multi-gym has the same stations. If you have trouble figuring out an exercise at an unsupervised hotel gym, look for a diagram on the side of the machine or ask another guest how to use it. (Don't worry about looking foolish; you'll never see these people again.) If you work out on enough of these contraptions, eventually you'll have the instincts to solve any multi-gym mystery.

Preworkout Briefing

Before each of the three workouts below, warm up with at least 5 minutes of easy cardiovascular exercise, such as walking your hotel steps or using a cardio machine. Do arm circles and shoulder rolls to warm up your upper body.

The Time-to-Kill Workout

This routine includes every exercise in the chapter. Most multi-gyms do not feature a calf station, so you may want to add the Heel Raise in Chapter 12. We also recommend adding a lower back exercise such as the Kneeling Back Extension or Alternating Back Extension in Chapter 12.

Sets: 1–3

Reps: 8–12

Rest: 30–60 seconds between exercises. Or do a circuit, moving from one exercise to the next without rest; in this case, lift slightly less weight than usual.

Lat Pulldown

Seated Chest Press Machine

Seated Row Machine

Lateral Cable Raise

Upright Row

Cable Biceps Curl

Triceps Pushdown

Seated Cable Crunch

Leg Press Machine

Seated Leg Extension

Standing Leg Curl Machine

The Timesaver Workout

This routine eliminates the extra back and shoulder exercises in the Time-to-Kill Workout.

Sets: 1–3

Reps: 8–12

Rest: 30 seconds or less

Lat Pulldown or Seated Row Machine

Seated Chest Press Machine

Lateral Cable Raise or Upright Row

Cable Biceps Curl

Triceps Pushdown

Seated Cable Crunch

Leg Press Machine

Standing Leg Curl Machine

Seated Leg Extension Machine

The Bare-Minimum Workout

This mini routine features four moves that, collectively, touch on all your major muscle groups other than your lower back and calves.

Sets: 1–3

Reps: 8–12

Rest: 30 seconds or less

Lat Pulldown

Seated Chest Press Machine

Leg Press Machine

Seated Cable Crunch

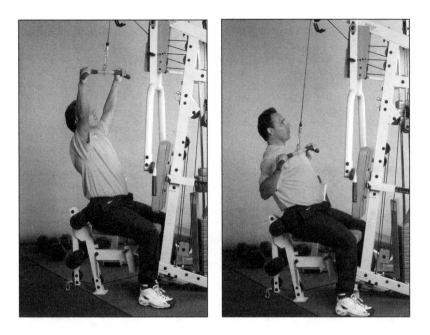

Muscles Worked: Middle Back, Biceps

Tip: Try this exercise with an underhand grip for variety.

The Setup: If the machine has thigh pads, adjust them so that your legs are firmly wedged underneath the pads with your knees bent and feet flat on the floor. Stand and grasp the bar with an overhand grip and your hands slightly wider than shoulder-width apart. Still grasping the bar, sit back down, with your arms extended overhead so you feel a slight stretch in your back. Lean back slightly from your hips.

The Action: Slowly pull the bar toward your chest, creating a slight arch in your back. Use your back muscles, rather than your arms, to do most of the pulling. Stop when the bar is about 3 inches from your chest, and slowly return to the starting position.

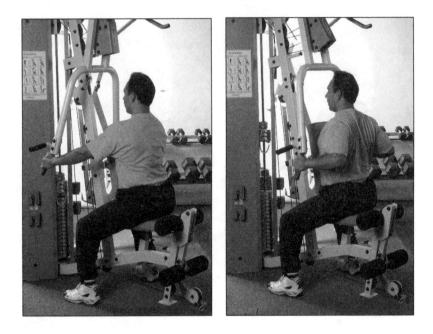

Muscles Worked: Middle and Upper Back, Biceps

Tip: Some multi-gyms feature a seated cable row, which targets the same muscle groups.

The Setup: Adjust the seat so that when you pull the handles back, your elbows form a 90-degree angle. Sit up straight with your chest against the pad and grasp the handles.

The Action: Maintaining perfect posture, pull the handles back until your elbows form a 90-degree angle. Squeeze your shoulder blades together so that your back muscles, not your biceps, do most of the work. Slowly straighten your arms, returning the handles to the starting position.

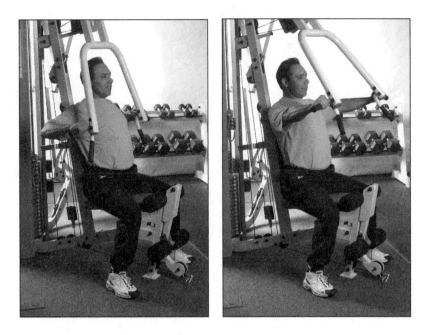

Muscles Worked: Chest, Triceps, Shoulders

Tip: Some multi-gyms feature a horizontal chest press.

The Setup: Adjust the seat height so that when you lower the weight, your arm is bent at a 90-degree angle. Sit up tall with your abdominals pulled in and your shoulders level. Grasp the handles and extend your arms until they are almost straight.

The Action: Maintaining good posture, slowly bend your elbows until your hands are in front of your chest and your arms form 90-degree angles. Contracting your chest muscles, push the handles forward until your elbows are straight but not locked. Then lower the handles to the starting position.

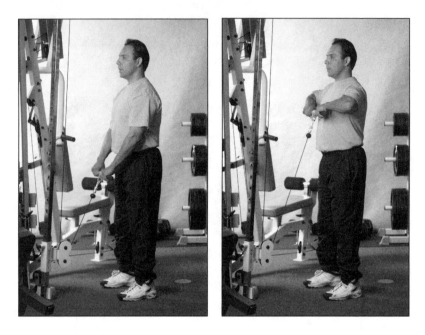

Muscles Worked: Upper Back, Shoulders

Tip: The traditional version of this exercise — lifting the bar to ear level — places excess stress on your shoulder joints, so perform this modified version.

The Setup: Attach a short bar to the low cable pulley. Grasp the bar with an overhand grip, and stand tall with your feet hip-width apart, shoulders back, abdominals pulled in, and arms outstretched.

The Action: Pull the bar up until your upper arms are parallel to the floor, no higher. As you slowly lower the bar, don't let the weight cause your shoulders to round forward.

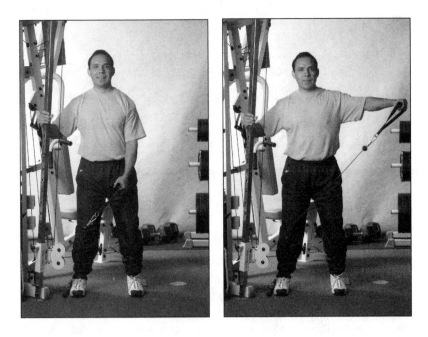

Muscles Worked: Shoulders

Tip: Don't lift your arms higher than parallel to the floor, a common mistake that places excess stress on the shoulder.

The Setup: Attach a handle to the low cable pulley, grasp the handle with your left hand, and stand with your right side to the machine so that the cable crosses your body diagonally. Let your left arm hang down in front of your thigh, palm facing back. Lightly grasp the pole with your right hand for support. Keep your feet hip-width apart, knees slightly bent, and abdominals pulled in.

The Action: Slowly lift your left arm out to the side until your arm is roughly parallel to the floor, elbow straight but not locked. Slowly lower your arm to the starting position, resisting gravity on the way down. Complete your set, turn around, grasp the handle with your right hand, and repeat.

CABLE BICEPS CURL

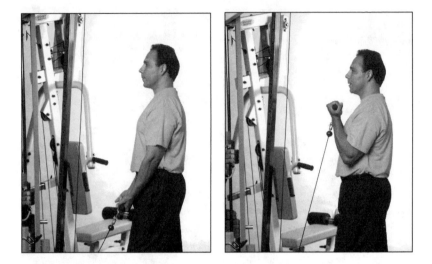

Muscles Worked: Biceps

Tip: If there isn't a short bar available, you can do this move with a rope.

The Setup: Attach a short bar to a low cable pulley. Grasp the bar with your hands shoulder-width apart, palms facing up. Stand tall with your feet hip-width apart and one foot ahead of the other, abdominals contracted, shoulders back, and arms hanging down to the sides. Feel a stretch in your biceps.

The Action: Keeping your elbows glued to your sides, curl the bar toward your shoulders without arching your back. Stop when your hands are a few inches from your shoulders and your biceps feel fatigued. Slowly lower the bar to the starting position. At the bottom, let the bar roll down your palm toward your fingers to allow for more of a biceps stretch. When you have completed the set, return the bar to the floor by bending at your knees and hips rather than leaning forward.

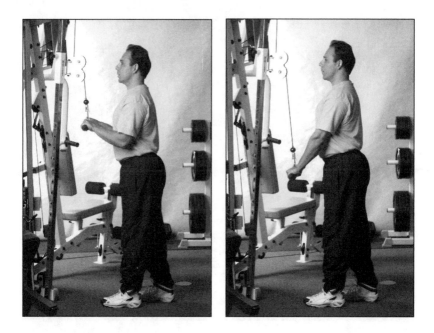

Muscle Worked: Triceps

Tip: Use the long bar used for the Lat Pulldown or the short bar used in the Cable Biceps Curl and Upright Row.

The Setup: Stand tall with your feet hip-width apart and one foot slightly ahead of the other, knees relaxed. If the seat is in your way, stand with your feet parallel to each other. Grasp the bar with an overhand grip and your hands shoulder-width apart, elbows against your sides. Place your forearms slightly above, parallel to the floor, and your wrists in line with your forearms, not bent. Pull your abdominals in and lean slightly forward at the waist.

The Action: Push the bar down, keeping your elbows close to your sides as you straighten your arms. Toward the bottom of the movement, allow your wrists to relax and bend upward. Then bend your arms, letting the bar slowly rise until your arms are slightly above parallel to the floor and your wrists are straight. Control the movement with your triceps, not momentum.

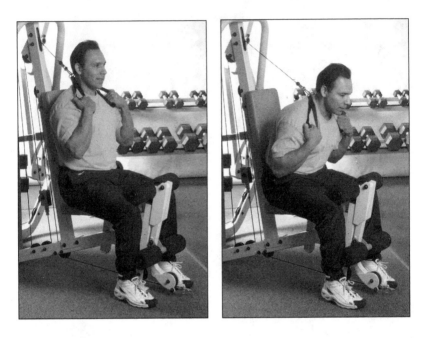

Muscles Worked: Abdominals

Tip: If your multi-gym doesn't have this station, lie on the floor and do the Rotational Crunch in Chapter 12.

The Setup: Attach a rope to the high cable pulley above the seat. Sit up tall with your abdominals tight and feet on the floor, and grasp the rope so that one hand is on either side of your neck, elbows pointing down.

The Action: Using your abdominal muscles, slowly curl your torso forward. Keep the movement subtle, lifting your back only 3 to 4 inches off the seat pad. Hold this position for a moment, keeping your abdominals contracted and your middle and upper back relaxed. Slowly return to the starting position, keeping tension on your abs.

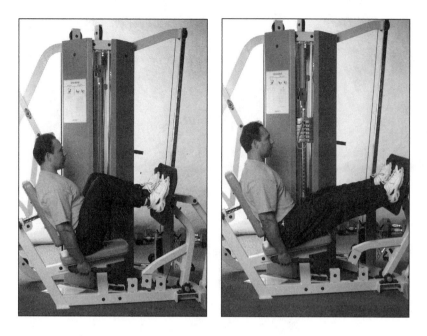

Muscles Worked: Quadriceps, Hamstrings, and Glutes

Tip: With some multi-gym leg press machines, you lie flat on your back. In this case, keep your head and neck on the pad, and don't raise your butt off the seat as you lower the weight, which can strain your lower back.

The Setup: Adjust the seat so that when your feet are on the plate, your knees are bent at a 90-degree angle. Place your feet hip-width apart with your toes pointing forward.

The Action: Push forward until your legs are almost straight. Bend your legs and slowly return to the starting position, making sure that your knees don't shoot in front of your toes.

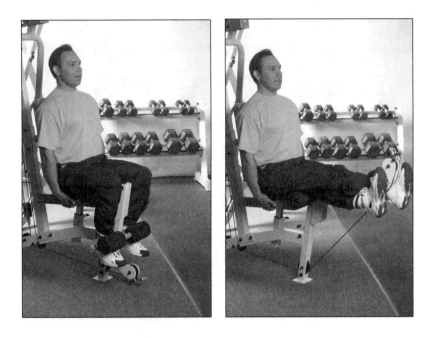

Muscle Worked: Quadriceps

The Setup: Adjust the machine so that you can sit comfortably against the back rest and your knees are lined up with the pivot point of the machine. If the ankle pad is adjustable, set it so that it's flush against your shins. Sit up straight with your back comfortably against the seat pad, legs hip-width apart, knees bent at 90 degrees, and abdominals pulled in.

The Action: Contracting your quadriceps, extend your legs until they are almost straight. Keep your feet relaxed under the pads. Slowly bend your knees, lowering the weight to the starting position.

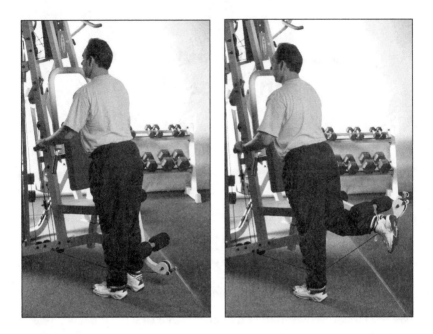

Muscle Worked: Hamstrings

Tip: If your multi-gym features a Lying Leg Curl, don't let your butt pop off the pad. This places stress on your lower back and minimizes the work done by your hamstrings.

The Setup: Adjust the seat so that your knees are in line with the axis point of the machine, your legs are hip-width apart, and your back rests comfortably against the pad. Stand tall with your abdominals pulled in and legs slightly bent.

The Action: Bend your knees, curling the pad as far underneath the seat as you can. Contracting your hamstrings, slowly straighten your legs to the starting position.

10

Dumbbell Routines for Any Occasion

Some people are so devoted to their dumbbell workouts that they will pack their steel weights in their suitcase and lug them on a business trip. Well, actually, there is probably only one person loopy enough to have done that: Liz Neporent, the New York City fitness consultant who designed the workouts in this chapter. "I packed a set of five-, eight- and twelve-pounders, thinking it would be no big deal since my luggage had wheels," says Neporent, who prefers the feel of cold, hard steel in her hands to that of rubber exercise tubing. "But the wheels broke at La Guardia, and I had to drag this load of cement through three airports. I was so sore and tired that I never even worked out."

Neporent hasn't packed dumbbells since, but she does use them whenever they are available. If you travel frequently, you may have noticed that many hotels don't offer dumbbells and barbells; they prefer to avoid the liability issues that may arise if a guest happens to drop a 40-pound weight on his toes — or on the toes of another guest. Still, plenty of hotel gyms do have free weights, which are a lot more versatile than weight machines. They also can be more comfortable to use because your body is not forced to follow a specific movement pattern.

> **Many hotels don't offer dumbbells and barbells; they prefer to avoid the liability issues that may arise if a guest happens to drop a 40-pound weight on his toes.**

This chapter demonstrates two dumbbell exercises for most of your major muscle groups so that you can mix and match for variety. (In hotel gyms, dumbbells are more common than barbells.) You'll also find four different workouts to choose from. A large repertoire of dumbbell exercises can be particularly helpful at small hotel gyms, where the weights may increase in large increments. For instance, on the road you may have to jump from 10 pounds to 15 pounds to 20 pounds, whereas your gym at home might have 12-pound and 17-pound dumbbells, too.

What the Heck Is 25 kg?

If you're mathematically challenged, one of the headaches of foreign travel is, of course, translating money from one currency to another. Just how expensive is that dress shirt for 175,000 yen? Well, if you're lifting weights abroad, you'll have to tax your brain with an additional calculation: translating kilograms to pounds, or vice versa. Just how heavy is that 25-kg dumbbell?

Most weight machines are American-made, so the weight plates are measured in pounds, but free weights outside the United States are often measured in kilograms. Making the conversion is important. At first glance, a 25-kilogram dumbbell may resemble the 45-pound weight you use at home, but it actually weighs 55 pounds — a fact you may not want to discover when you have two of these overhead in the middle of your Incline Chest Fly.

One kilogram equals 2.2 pounds; one pound equals .45 of a kilogram. To save you trouble of doing math in your head, here's a handy chart to help you make the conversions.

Kilograms	Pounds	Pounds	Kilograms
2	4.4	3	1.4
3	6.6	5	2.3
4	8.8	8	3.6
5	11	10	4.5
6	13.2	12	5.4
8	17.6	15	6.8
9	19.8	20	9.1
10	22	25	11.4
12	26.4	30	13.6
15	33	35	15.9
20	44	40	18.2
25	55	45	20.5
45	66	50	22.7

If your hotel gym doesn't have the weight you need for a particular exercise, pick an alternative move that allows you to use more weight. For instance, if you don't have a dumbbell light enough for the Triceps Kickback, choose the Overhead Triceps Press, which you probably can do with a weight twice as heavy. If there's no dumbbell in the right range, err on the lighter side and do a few more repetitions. Or do what Liz Neporent now does: Fish out that rubber tube in your suitcase.

Preworkout Briefing

The workouts in this chapter don't include exercises for your abdominals or lower back because these muscles are best worked without weights. To each routine, add the Rotational Crunch, an abdominal exercise that you can perform on the floor, either at the gym or back in your room. To strengthen your lower back, do the Kneeling Back Extension, using your hotel bed, or a version performed on the floor. We also suggest adding the Heel Raise, which you can perform while holding a dumbbell. (Skip ahead to Chapter 12 for descriptions of all of these exercises.)

Before any of the dumbbell workouts, warm up with at least 5 minutes of cardiovascular exercise, such a walking briskly around the hotel, climbing stairs, or using a cardio machine. Do arm circles and shoulder rolls to warm up your upper body.

The Time-to-Kill Workout

This routine includes all of the exercises in this chapter, allowing you to work your major muscle groups from different angles.

Sets: 1–3
Reps: 8–12
Rest: 30–60 seconds

One-Arm Dumbbell Row	Alternating Biceps Curl
Dumbbell Pullover	Concentration Curl
Dumbbell Chest Press	Overhead Triceps Press
Incline Chest Fly	Triceps Kickback
Dumbbell Shoulder Press	Dumbbell Squat
Rear Delt Fly	Dumbbell Lunge

Timesaver Workouts

Both Timesaver Workouts hit your major muscle groups. Timesaver Workout 1 features exercises that typically require heavier weights than the equivalent moves in Timesaver Workout 2. For instance, when working your chest muscles, you tend to use more weight with the Dumbbell Chest Press than you do with the Incline Chest Fly. The Dumbbell Shoulder Press requires heavier weights than the Rear Delt Fly, and so on. We've divided the exercises in this way so that if you don't have a dumbbell that is the right weight for one exercise, you can quickly figure out which substitute to try.

Sets: 1–3
Reps: 8–12
Rest: None (Do a circuit. See Chapter 8.)

Timesaver Workout 1

One-Arm Dumbbell Row
Dumbbell Chest Press
Dumbbell Shoulder Press
Alternating Biceps Curl
Overhead Triceps Press
Dumbbell Squat

Timesaver Workout 2

Dumbbell Pullover
Incline Chest Fly
Rear Delt Fly
Concentration Curl
Triceps Kickback
Dumbbell Lunge

The Bare-Minimum Workout

Do this routine when you only have 10 minutes to work out. Each of the exercises works more than one muscle group.

Sets: 1–3
Reps: 8–12
Rest: 30 seconds

One-Arm Dumbbell Row
Dumbbell Chest Press
Dumbbell Squat or Lunge

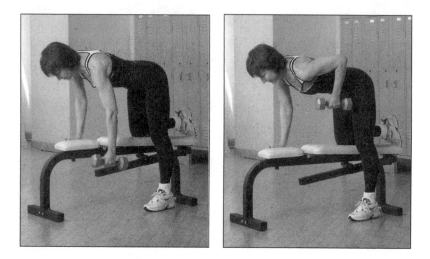

Muscles Worked: Upper Back, Biceps, Shoulders

Tip: This is a back exercise, not an arm exercise, so focus on pulling from your back muscles rather than just moving your arm up and down.

The Setup: Holding a dumbbell in your left hand, stand to the left of a weight bench. Place your right shin and right hand on top of the bench for support. Let your left arm hang down and a bit forward, palm facing in. Pull your abdominals in and bend forward from your hips so your back is naturally arched and roughly parallel to the floor, and your left knee is slightly bent. Tilt your chin toward your chest so your neck is in line with the rest of your spine.

The Action: Pull your left arm up until your upper arm is parallel to the floor, your hand brushes against your waist, and your elbow points to the ceiling. Don't let your back sag toward the floor or hunch up. Slowly lower the weight back down. When you've completed the set, switch sides.

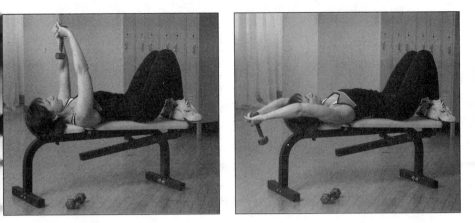

Muscles Worked: Middle Back, Chest, Shoulders, Biceps, Abdominals

Tip: Use a relatively light weight for this exercise to avoid straining your abdominals.

The Setup: Holding a single dumbbell securely with both hands, lie on your back with your feet up the bench or flat on the floor (whichever is more comfortable), arms directly over your shoulders. Turn your palms up so that one end of the dumbbell is resting in the gap between your palms and the other end is hanging down above your face. Pull your abdominals in but make sure your back is relaxed and arched naturally.

The Action: Keeping your elbows slightly bent, lower the weight until the bottom of the dumbbell is directly behind your head. Focus on initiating the movement from the outer wings of your upper back rather than simply bending and straightening your arms. Pull the dumbbell back overhead, maintaining the same slight bend in your elbows.

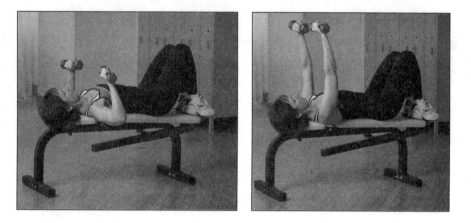

Muscles Worked: Chest, Shoulders, Triceps

Tip: If you perform this exercise on an incline bench, use less weight.

The Setup: Lie on a bench with a dumbbell in each hand, palms facing up, and your feet on the bench or flat on the floor. Press the dumbbells up so that your arms are directly over your shoulders. Pull your abdominals in, and tilt your chin toward your chest.

The Action: Lower the dumbbells down and a bit to the side until your elbows are slightly below your shoulders. Press the weights back up. Don't let your shoulder blades rise off the bench, and don't lock your elbows at the top of the motion.

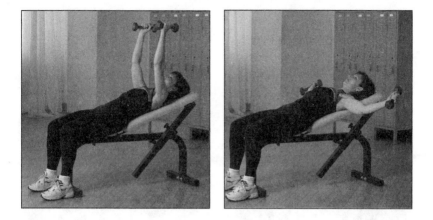

Muscles Worked: Chest, Shoulders

Tip: If you perform the Chest Fly on a flat bench, you probably can use a bit more weight.

The Setup: Adjust the bench so that it is moderately inclined. Holding a dumbbell in each hand, lie on the bench with your feet flat on the floor. Press the weights directly above your chest, arms slightly bent and palms facing each other. Tuck your chin to your chest to align your neck with the rest of your spine. Maintain your natural back posture, neither arched nor flattened.

The Action: Spreading your arms apart so that your elbows travel down and to the sides, lower the weights until your elbows are just below your shoulders. Imagine you have a barrel lying on your chest and you have to keep your arms wide to reach around it. Maintain a constant bend in your elbows as you lift the dumbbells back up.

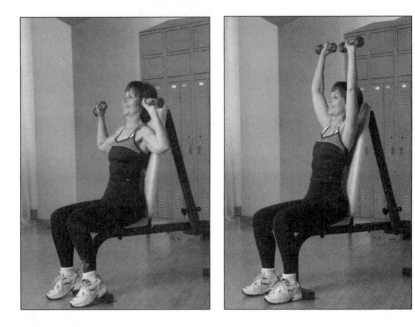

Muscles Worked: Shoulders

Tip: If you don't have a bench with a straight back, you can perform this exercise while standing with your knees slightly bent.

The Setup: Hold a dumbbell in each hand and sit on a bench with back support. Plant your feet firmly on the floor and about hip-width apart. Bend your elbows and raise your upper arms to shoulder height so the dumbbells are at ear level, palms facing forward. Pull your abdominals in so there is a slight gap between the small of your back and the bench. Rest the back of your head against the pad.

The Action: Push the dumbbells up and in until the ends of the weights almost touch directly over your head. At the top, keep your elbows relaxed rather than locked. Then lower the dumbbells back to ear level.

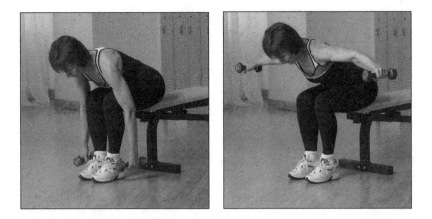

Muscles Worked: Rear Shoulders, Upper Back

Tip: Lean forward from your hips rather than rounding your back.

The Setup: Hold a dumbbell in each hand and sit on the edge of a bench. Lean forward so your upper back is flat and parallel to the floor. (If you can, support your chest against your knees.) Let your arms hang down so your palms face each other with the weights behind your calves, directly under your knees. Tuck your chin toward your chest and pull in your abdominals.

The Action: Lift your arms up and out to the sides, bending your elbows a few inches as you go until your elbows are level with your shoulders. Squeeze your shoulder blades together as you lift. Slowly lower your arms back down.

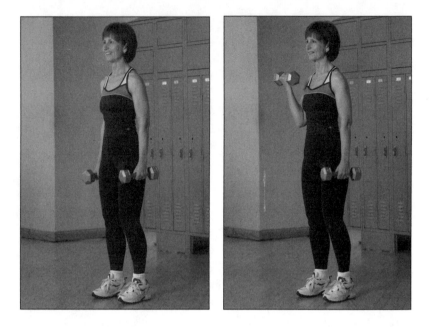

Muscles Worked: Biceps

Tip: To save time, perform this exercise with both arms at once, starting with your palms facing forward.

The Setup: Hold a dumbbell in each hand and stand with your feet hip-width apart. Let your arms hang down at your sides, palms facing in. Pull your abdominals in, stand straight, and keep your knees relaxed.

The Action: Curl your right arm close to your shoulder, twisting your palm as you go so that it faces the front of your shoulder at the top of the movement. Slowly lower the weight back down, then repeat with your left arm.

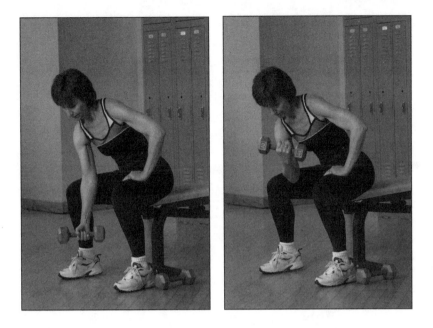

Muscles Worked: Biceps

Tip: As you lift the weight, don't cheat by leaning away from your arm to get better leverage.

The Setup: Hold a dumbbell in your right hand and sit on the edge of a bench with your feet a few inches wider than your hips. Lean forward from your hips and place your right elbow against the inside of your right thigh, just behind your knee. The weight should hang down near the inside of your ankle. Place your left palm on top of your left thigh.

The Action: Bend your arm and curl the dumbbell almost, but not quite, up to your shoulder. Then straighten your arm to lower the weight back down. Complete your reps with your right arm before switching sides.

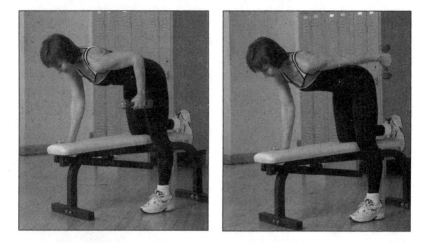

Muscles Worked: Triceps

Tip: Don't let your upper arm move or let your shoulder drop below your waist.

The Setup: Hold a dumbbell in your left hand and stand to the left of your weight bench. Place your right shin and right hand on the bench. Lean forward at your hips until your upper body is at a 45-degree angle to the floor. Bend your left elbow so your upper arm is parallel to the floor, your forearm is perpendicular to it, and your palm faces in. Keep your elbow close to your waist. Pull your abdominals in and relax your knees.

The Action: Keeping your upper arm still, straighten your left arm behind you until your entire arm is parallel to the floor and the dumbbell points down. Slowly bend your arm to lower the weight. After you complete the set, switch sides.

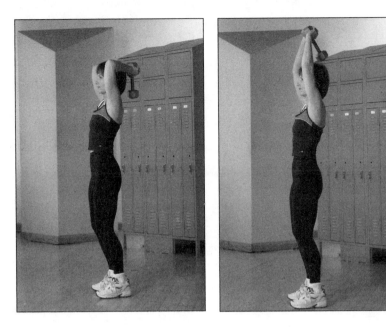

Muscles Worked: Triceps

Tip: You can also perform this exercise while seated on the edge of a bench with your feet flat on the floor.

The Setup: Stand tall with your feet hip-width apart, abdominals contracted, knees slightly bent, holding one dumbbell with both hands. Lift the weight directly overhead, then shift your hand position so that the dumbbell slides down a bit, your palms face the ceiling, and the weight is resting between your thumbs. Keeping your elbows stationary and abdominals tight, slowly lower the weight behind your head.

The Action: Maintaining your elbow position, press the dumbbell up until it is directly overhead and your palms face the ceiling. Lower the weight back down.

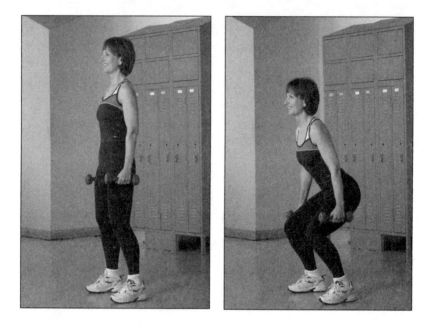

Muscles Worked: Glutes, Quadriceps, and Hamstrings

Tip: To help maintain your balance, keep your head up and your eyes focused in front of you. Don't look down or shift your body weight forward.

The Setup: Hold a dumbbell in each hand with your arms hanging down at your sides. Stand with your feet hip-width apart and your weight slightly back on your heels. Pull your abdominals in and stand up tall with your chest lifted.

The Action: Sit back and down, as if you're lowering yourself into a chair. Lower as far as you can without leaning your upper body more than a few inches forward. Don't lower any farther than the point at which your thighs are parallel to the floor, and don't let your knees shoot out in front of your toes. Once you feel your upper body fold forward over your thighs, straighten your legs and stand back up.

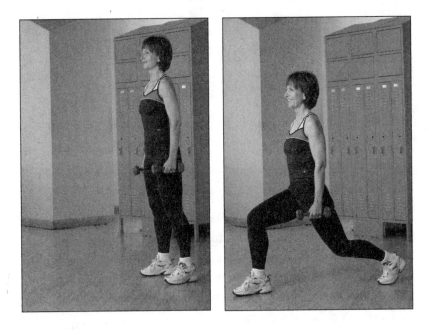

Muscles Worked: Glutes, Quadriceps, Hamstrings, Calves

Tip: If you're new to this exercise, do the Tubing Split Lunge (see Chapter 11) but with a dumbbell in each hand rather than a tube.

The Setup: Hold a dumbbell in each hand with your arms hanging down at your sides. Stand with your feet hip-width apart and your weight back a bit on your heels. Pull your abdominals in and stand up tall with your chest lifted.

The Action: Take a giant step forward with your right foot, leading with your heel. As your foot touches the floor, bend both knees until your right thigh is parallel to the floor and your left thigh is perpendicular to it. Your left heel will lift off the floor. Don't let your right knee travel past your toes. Press off the ball of your foot and step back to the starting position. Complete all reps with your right leg before switching sides.

11

Band on the Run: A Quick Tubing Workout

If you're accustomed to hoisting hunks of steel and operating heavy machinery at the gym, you may wonder whether you can actually challenge your muscles with a dinky rubber exercise tube. Well, you can.

With a thick enough tube and the right body position, just about anyone can get a decent workout. Florida trainer Troy DeMond managed to convince perhaps one of the world's most skeptical audiences: a group of customs agents at the airport in Sao Paulo, Brazil.

> **With a thick enough tube and the right body position, just about anyone can get a decent workout.**

DeMond had packed 200 tubes to bring to a fitness convention. When customs officials opened his suitcase and discovered the mysterious contents, they began yanking on the tubes and interrogating DeMond in Portuguese. "It was very nerve-wracking," DeMond recalls. "They were probably thinking there was cocaine in the tubing." In an attempt at self-preservation, DeMond grabbed one of the tubes and began demonstrating biceps curls and lateral raises. "Once they got the gist, five of them started doing the exercises with me," DeMond says. The agents found the tubes to their liking — so much so that they insisted on keeping them. "Hey," DeMond says, "I wasn't going to argue."

The workout in this chapter, designed by DeMond, uses a tube with handles on each end. You also can perform these exercises with a flat band, although it'll be less comfortable for your hands. You can learn additional tubing exercises from a video or a manual, such as those mentioned in Chapter 2.

If you don't have access to a gym, a tube is an invaluable tool for maintaining your strength on the road. You can perform tubing exercises anywhere — in a hotel room, a park, even a tent. Of course, you can also do them at the airport. You certainly won't be the first one to have tried.

Tubing Safety Tips

Pulling on exercise tubing isn't exactly a risky activity. Still, to keep the tube from snapping into your face — and to give your muscles the best challenge — follow these important guidelines.

- Check for holes or worn spots in the tubing. Replace the tube if you see any tears.

- Do your workout on carpeting, wood floors, or grass — anywhere but asphalt or cement. Abrasive surfaces can tear your tube.

- Wear comfortable, supportive athletic shoes, not sandals or dress shoes.

- Make sure the tubing is secured underfoot before you begin each exercise.

- Maintain good posture throughout each exercise: Keep your knees slightly bent, your abdominal muscles pulled in, and your chest expanded.

- Perform the exercises in a slow and controlled manner, to work against resistance both when you pull on the tube and when you return to the starting position.

The Three Starting Positions

You can anchor the tubing to the floor in three different ways. The position you choose for each exercise will depend on your strength and the specific demands of that exercise. If you can't complete 8 reps for an exercise, use an easier foot position or a thinner tube. If 12 reps is too easy, choose a more difficult foot position or a thicker tube.

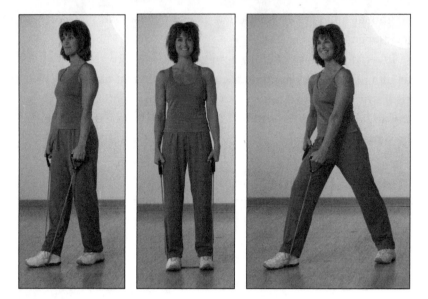

- **Staggered Stance:** Stand with one foot on the tubing and the other foot slightly behind. This position offers the least amount of resistance.

- **Moderate Stance:** Stand with both feet on the tubing slightly less than hip-width apart.

- **Wide Stance:** Stand with both feet on the tubing wider than hip-width apart. This stance is the most challenging.

Preworkout Briefing

The workouts in this chapter don't include exercises for your abdominals or lower back because these muscles are best worked without equipment. To each routine, add the Bedside Crunch or the Rotational Crunch, both in Chapter 12. To strengthen your lower back, do the Kneeling Back Extension, using your hotel bed, or a version performed on the floor, the Alternating Back Extension, also both in the next chapter.

Before each workout, warm up with at least 5 minutes of easy cardiovascular exercise, such as walking your hotel stairs, walking briskly down the hallways, or doing the calisthenics in Chapter 6. Practice all of the exercises without the tubing until you master the motion.

The Timesaver Tubing Workout

This routine includes one exercise for each upper-body muscle group and two exercises that hit the main muscle groups in your lower body.

Sets: 1–3
Reps: 8–12
Rest: 30–60 seconds. Or eliminate the rest and do a circuit.
  (See Chapter 8.)

Tubing Row
Tubing Chest Cross
Tubing Shoulder Press
Tubing Biceps Curl

Tubing Triceps Extension
Tubing Squat
Tubing Split Lunge

The Bare-Minimum Tubing Workout

This routine hits your major muscle groups with the fewest tubing exercises possible.

Sets: 1–3
Reps: 8–12
Rest: None

Tubing Row
Tubing Chest Cross
Tubing Shoulder Press
Tubing Split Lunge

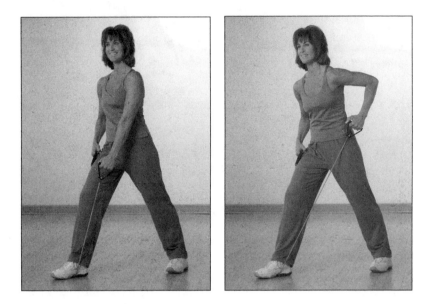

Muscles Worked: Middle Back, Biceps

Tip: Always keep your nonworking hand on your thigh for back support.

The Setup: Holding one handle in each hand, step on the tube with your right foot. Place your left foot back in a staggered lunge and your right hand on your right thigh. Shorten the tubing so it's taut. Your left palm should face the inner thigh of your right leg. Bend slightly forward from the hip.

The Action: Move your left elbow up behind your back, as if you're about to start a lawn mower. Slowly lower to the starting position. Complete the set, then switch sides.

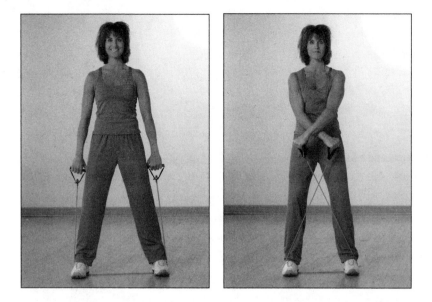

Muscles Worked: Chest

Tip: Keep your arms relatively straight so your chest muscles get a sufficient challenge.

The Setup: With one handle in each hand, stand with your feet wider than hip-width apart on the tubing, knees slightly bent, arms relaxed, palms facing back.

The Action: Cross your hands in front of your body until your wrists or elbows cross. Your hands should remain facing your thighs with your knuckles pointing down.

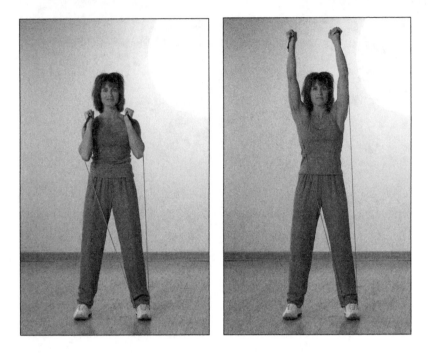

Muscles Worked: Shoulders

Tip: As you raise your hands, keep your abs tight and don't arch your back.

The Setup: Stand with your feet hip-width apart but with only one foot on the tube, hands at shoulder height, palms facing each other, elbows tucked in and pointing down.

The Action: Press your hands up to ceiling, finishing with your hands directly above your shoulders, palms facing each other, as if you're signaling a touchdown.

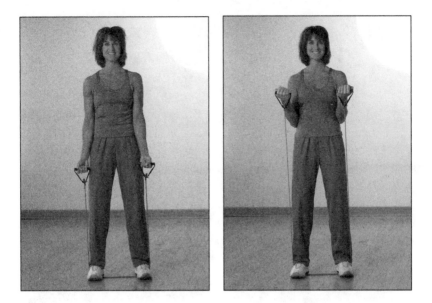

Muscles Worked: Biceps

Tip: Make sure your band is plenty taut at the top of the movement.

The Setup: Start in either the moderate or wide stance, with your arms relaxed at your sides. Grasp the handles with your palms facing forward.

The Action: Keeping your elbows tight against your sides, curl your hands up until your palms face your body and your elbows point to the ground.

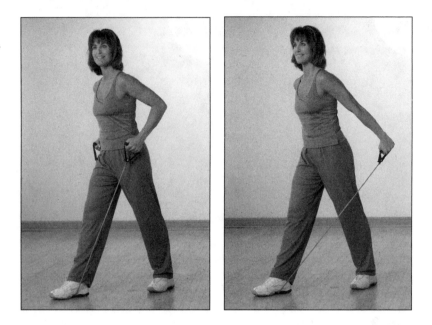

Muscles Worked: Triceps

Tip: As you perform this move, imagine that your lower arms are windshield wipers.

The Setup: Stand in the staggered stance with either foot on the tube, and grasp the handles, arms hanging down, palms facing the side of your thighs. Raise your upper arms and cock your elbows at a 90-degree angle behind you.

The Action: Keeping your elbows still, push your hands back, straightening your arms to a nearly locked position. Complete the set, then switch sides.

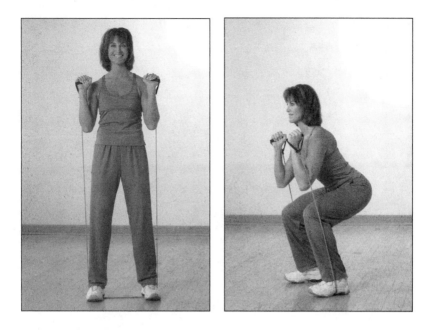

Muscles Worked: Quadriceps, Hamstrings, Glutes

Tip: To master the mechanics, place a chair behind you for the first few repetitions.

The Setup: Stand with your feet hip-width apart on the tubing, holding the handles at shoulder height, elbows pointing down. The tubing should be taut.

The Action: With your abdominals tight and chest lifted, sit back as if you're about to plant yourself on a chair. Squat as low as you can but no lower than the point at which your thighs are parallel to the floor. Make sure your knees don't shoot ahead of your toes. Hold the squat for 2 seconds, pressing your feet through the floor, then stand back up.

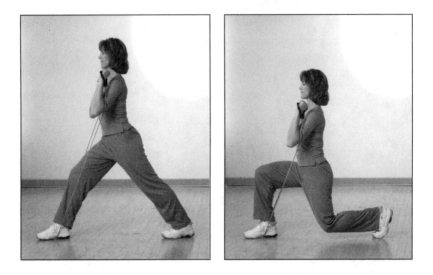

Muscles Worked: Quadriceps, Hamstrings, Glutes

Tip: To target your quadriceps most effectively, move your torso straight up and down rather than forward or back.

The Setup: Place your right foot on the center of the tube, and stand with your feet hip-width apart. Hold the handles at shoulder height so that the tubing is taut and your elbows are pointing down. Step straight back with your left foot and bend your left knee slightly. Imagine that there are two train tracks and you have one foot on each.

The Action: With your abdominals tight and chest lifted, lower your torso so that your tailbone is pointing straight down, your left leg is slightly bent, and you're up on the ball of your left foot. If you can't see your toes, you've lunged too far forward. Push back up to the starting position. Perform all repetitions on one side before switching sides.

12

The Last Resort: Strength Training Without Equipment

There isn't a dumbbell or weight machine in the vicinity, and you didn't pack an exercise tube. What now? No, we do not recommend heading to the hotel bar for a set of biceps curls with a bottle of Amstel Light. You can actually get a decent strength workout right in your hotel room, by using your own body weight as resistance and working slowly against gravity.

Just keep in mind that strength training without equipment has its limitations. You can work your abs, lower back, chest, and triceps quite well, but your upper back and biceps muscles will get short shrift. These muscle groups are best worked with pulling movements, which are tough to manage without at least rubber tubing (although you could do the One-Arm Dumbbell in Chapter 10 with a heavy briefcase or small, weighted duffel bag). Your butt and thigh muscles also can be difficult to strengthen without equipment because they are naturally quite strong. However, you can probably create a sufficient challenge if you perform the exercises in this chapter while wearing a backpack. Just remember to center the objects in your pack.

> You can actually get a decent strength workout right in your hotel room, by using your own body weight as resistance and working slowly against gravity.

The workouts in this chapter were designed by Los Angeles trainer Ken Alan, who is well acquainted with the benefits—and potential hazards—of strength training in a hotel room. Once, while on business in Cleveland, Alan was performing an isometric leg press in his hotel closet, with his back firmly against one wall and his feet pressed up against the other. When he pushed forward, his feet flew right through the drywall and his back left a dent in the wall behind him. "I thought the whole room was caving in," recalls Alan, who placed a trash bin against the hole and quietly checked out of the hotel.

Rest assured that the exercises shown here won't cause any property damage. They'll simply strengthen your muscles, provided that you pay close attention to your technique and perform them very slowly. When you have no equipment, shift your focus from quantity—how much weight you can squat or how many pushups you can do—to the quality of your movements. This workout emphasizes your postural muscles: your abdominals, lower back muscles, and glutes. These muscles are particularly important for travelers (see Chapter 8), but they often get neglected when there are hunks of steel to throw around.

Preworkout Briefing

As usual, we recommend that you perform 8 to 12 repetitions per set. However, because it's difficult to adjust the resistance with some of these exercises—you can't just pick up a heavier weight—you may have to relax that rule. If you can perform more than 8 to 12 repetitions of an exercise, choose a more difficult version of that move. If you're still not sufficiently challenged, increase the repetitions until you hit 20. If you're a beginner, you may have to stop at as few as 4 repetitions for some exercises and rest as long as 90 seconds between sets.

Keep in mind that these workouts do not include exercises for your middle and upper back or biceps, so at some point on your travels, try to find a gym where you can work these muscle groups or buy a tube. (You can find several middle and upper back and biceps exercises in Chapters 9 through 11.) Before this workout, warm up with at least 5 minutes of easy cardiovascular exercise, such as climbing your hotel stairs, jogging down the hallway, or doing the calisthenics in Chapter 6.

The Time-to-Kill Hotel-Room Workout

This routine, which emphasizes the abdominal and lower back muscles, includes all of the exercises in this chapter.

Sets: 1–3
Reps: 4–20 (See Preworkout Briefing.)
Rest: 30–90 seconds

Pushup	Alternating Back Extension
Triceps Dip	Alternating Back Extension
Bedside Crunch	One-Legged Lunge
Rotational Crunch	Traveling Lunge
Kneeling Back Extension	Heel Raise

The Timesaver Hotel-Room Workout

This routine is a pared-down version of the Time-to-Kill Workout.

Sets: 1–3
Reps: 4–20 (See Preworkout Briefing.)
Rest: 30–90 seconds

Pushup	Alternating Back Extension
Triceps Dip	One-Legged Lunge
Rotational Crunch	Traveling Lunge

The Bare-Minimum Hotel-Room Workout

This routine doesn't come close to working your entire body but does include four challenging exercises that probably aren't part of your regular strength routine.

Sets: 1–3
Reps: 4–20 (See Preworkout Briefing.)
Rest: 30–90 seconds

Pushup
Rotational Crunch
Kneeling Back Extension
One-Legged Lunge

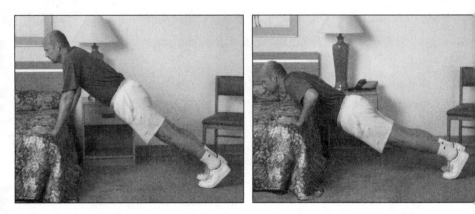

Muscles Worked: Chest, Shoulders, Triceps

Tip: This is the easiest of the three pushup versions. If it's too challenging, start on your knees about 18 inches from the bed and lean forward with your palms on the edge of the bed.

The Setup: Place your palms on the edge of the bed slightly wider than your shoulders with your fingers pointed forward. Scoot your body back so that your arms and legs are straight, with your feet slightly apart.

The Action: Contract your abdominal muscles to keep your torso still and tuck your chin slightly to keep your neck and head in alignment. Bend your elbows and lower your body until your elbows form a 90-degree angle, no farther. Your chest need not touch the floor or bed. Slowly push up until your elbows are almost straight.

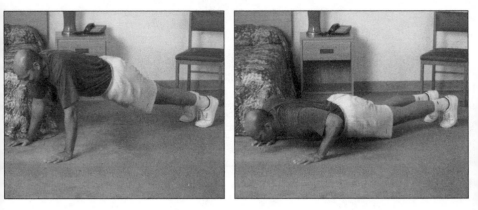

Muscles Worked: Chest, Shoulders, Triceps

Tip: Perform this move slowly enough and with such stellar control that you cannot do more than 15 to 20 repetitions.

The Setup: Lie facedown on the floor with your legs straight out behind you and slightly apart. Place your palms slightly wider than your shoulders, fingers pointed forward. Straighten your arms and lift your body so you're balanced on your palms and the underside of your toes.

The Action: Contract your abdominals to keep your torso still and tuck your chin slightly to keep your neck and head in alignment. Bend your elbows and lower your body until your elbows form a 90-degree angle, no farther. Your chest need not touch the floor. Slowly push up until your elbows are almost straight.

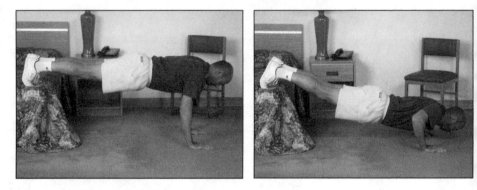

Muscles Worked: Chest, Shoulders, Triceps

Tip: Be sure you are proficient at the Military Pushup before attempting this very advanced move.

The Setup: Facing away from the bed, place your hands on the floor slightly wider than your shoulders, fingers pointed forward and arms straight. Place your feet on the bed with your legs straight and slightly apart.

The Action: Contract your abdominals to keep your towso still and tuck your chin slightly to keep your neck and head in alignment. Bend your elbows and lower your body until your elbows form a 90-degree angle, no farther. Your chest need not touch the floor. Slowly push up until your elbows are almost straight.

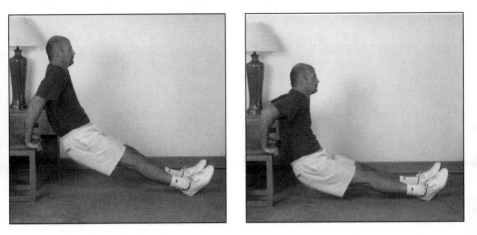

Muscles Worked: Triceps, Shoulders

Tip: If this exercise is too challenging, bend your knees at a right angle.

The Setup: Place a sturdy chair against the bed or wall. With your back to the chair, place your hands on the seat, fingers forward and wrapped over the edge. Supporting yourself with your arms, scoot your legs forward until they are straight and your butt is away from the chair seat.

The Action: Slowly bend your elbows to lower your torso. When your elbows are bent between 45 and 90 degrees, push back up until your arms are almost straight.

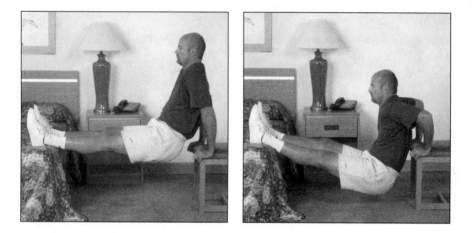

Muscles Worked: Triceps, Shoulders

Tip: For more of a challenge, place some weight on your lap, like a carry-on bag. Avoid this exercise if you have shoulder problems.

The Setup: Place a sturdy chair 3 to 4 feet from the bed and facing it. (Other options: Use two chairs facing each other or one chair facing a hard suitcase.) Place your hands on the seat, fingers forward and wrapped over the edge. Place your feet on the chair seat with your legs straight, supporting yourself with your arms. Move your torso toward your feet a bit so that you clear the edge of the bed when doing the exercise.

The Action: Slowly bend your elbows to lower your torso. When your elbows are bent between 45 and 90 degrees, push back up until your arms are almost straight.

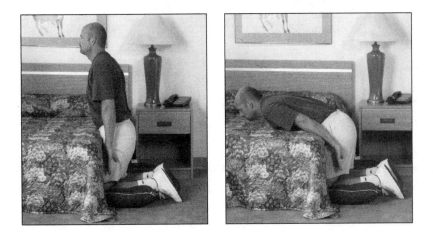

Muscles Worked: Lower Back, Glutes

Tip: To make this exercise more difficult, place your arms out to the side at shoulder level or overhead in a Superman position.

The Setup: Kneel on a pillow or folded towel facing the bed. Bend forward at the hip until your torso and forehead are facedown on the bed. Place your arms by the sides of your torso, palms up. If necessary, place another pillow under your knees to elevate yourself so your hips sit at the edge of the bed.

The Action: Contract your hamstrings, glutes, and lower back muscles, then take 4 to 8 seconds to lift your torso until you are vertical. Keep your hips on the edge of the bed at all times. If necessary, use your hands for assistance by pressing them lightly on the bed. Keep your shoulders down and slightly back, and maintain a natural arch in your lower back, throughout the exercise, rather than rounding it. Keep your head and neck aligned with your spine by slightly tucking your chin. Take 6 seconds to lower your torso back down to the bed. Rest for 2 seconds and repeat.

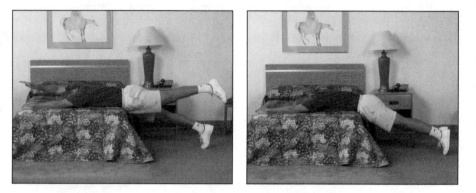

Muscles Worked: Lower Back, Rear Shoulders, Glutes

Tip: You also can perform this move while lying on the floor with your arms and legs straight. Lift your right arm and left leg a few inches off the floor, stretching as much as possible. Then lower and switch sides.

The Setup: Kneel facing the bed. Bend forward at the hip, and rest your torso and forehead on the bed. Place your arms on the bed, above your head in a Superman position. Walk your feet away from the bed and extend your knees until they are off the floor. You should be on your toes, supporting the weight of your legs. If needed, place a pillow at the edge of the bed under your abdomen for comfort.

The Action: Simultaneously lift your right arm up and left leg as high as you can. Hold for a moment, keeping your head and neck in alignment on the bed. Your hips should remain on the bed throughout the exercise. Lower slowly, then lift your left arm and right leg. Alternate sides, taking a full 8 to 10 seconds for each repetition.

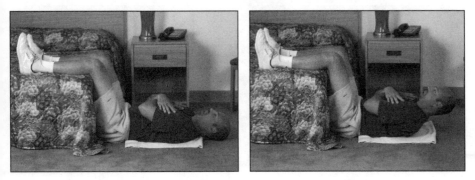

Muscles Worked: Abdominals

Tip: Alter your arm position to make the exercise easier or more difficult. The easiest position: Rest your arms by your sides. For more of a challenge, cross them over your chest or place them behind your head, hands lightly clasped and fingers interlaced. The toughest position: Extend your hands overhead.

The Setup: Fold a bath towel in half, and place it on the floor about 4 inches away from the bed. Lie on your back on the towel, and scoot close to the bed so you can drape your legs on the bed. Rest your hamstrings against the side of the bed and your lower legs on top of the bed.

The Action: Tighten your abdominals, as if someone's about to punch you in the belly, and use these muscles to lift your shoulders and upper back off the floor a few inches off the floor. Hold for a moment, and make a serious effort to pull in your gut and make your navel actually move downward. Hold for 2 seconds, then slowly lower your torso to the starting position, keeping your navel drawn in. Relax for a moment, then repeat, taking an intense 5 to 8 seconds for every rep.

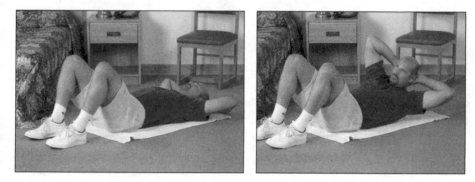

Muscles Worked: Adominals (including obliques)

Tip: Concentrate on rotating from your middle rather than simply moving your elbows toward your knees.

The Setup: Lie on your back with your knees bent and feet hip-width apart and flat on the floor. Place your hands behind your head, fingers slightly clasped. Your elbows should be out to the side but rounded slightly inward.

The Action: As you curl your head, neck, and shoulder blades off the floor, twist your torso slightly to the left, bringing your right shoulder toward your right knee. (Your elbow will not come close to touching your knee.) Make a purposeful effort to pull your abdominals in, then lower your back down. Alternate sides as you complete the set.

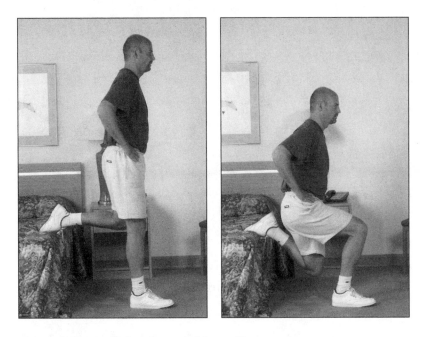

Muscles Worked: Quadriceps, Glutes, Hamstrings

Tip: Using the bed not only makes this move tougher than the traditional version of this exercise (shown in Chapter 11 with a tube) but also helps develop your ability to balance.

The Setup: Stand 2 feet from the bed, with your back to it, your feet a bit wider than your hips, and your toes facing forward. Carefully place your left foot behind you on the bed, the top of your foot facing down. (Easier version: Place your left foot on the floor behind you.) Stand tall on your right leg, foot pointed forward, abdominals pulled in, shoulders relaxed, hands on your hips. If you're wobbly, place your hand on the wall or on a chair beside you for balance.

The Action: Slowly bend your right knee, lowering as far as you can while still controlling the movement. Don't lean forward as you lower. You won't bend as far down as you would doing a squat. Keep your right knee aligned over your right toes and keep your torso and head upright. Push back up to the starting position.

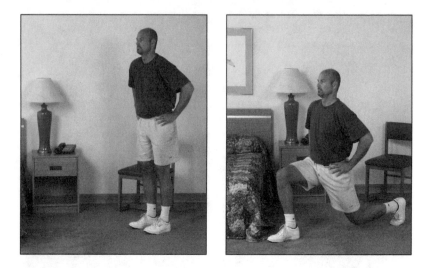

Muscles Worked: Glutes, Quadriceps, Inner and Outer Thighs, Hamstrings

Tip: You'll have to venture into the hallway, unless you're staying in the presidential suite. Warm up well before attempting the Traveling Lunge and, if you feel any knee pain, perform the squats instead. (Do the Dumbbell Squat in Chapter 10 without the dumbbells.) To make the exercise even tougher, wear a backpack.

The Setup: Stand with your feet hip-width apart, knees slightly bent, hands on your hips, toes pointed forward, abdominals pulled in, shoulders down and pulled slightly back. Look straight ahead.

The Action: Take a big step forward with your right foot, bending both knees. As you place your right foot on the floor, lift onto the toes of your left foot. Keep your left leg bent, balancing in the bottom position for a moment. Your right knee and toes should point forward. If your knee shoots beyond your toes, step forward a bit more on the next rep. Contract the muscles in your right leg to stand back up and immediately step forward with your left foot. Continue alternating right and left legs as you lunge forward 12 to 30 steps. As you step, maintain an upright posture, and keep your feet hip-width apart.

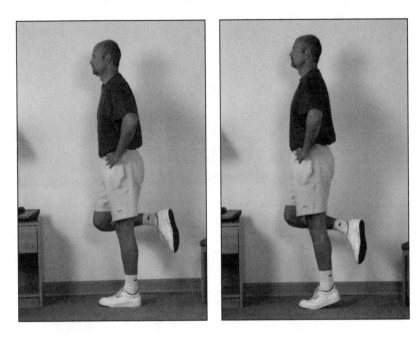

Muscles Worked: Calves

Tip: Beginners may want to do this exercise with both feet at the same time.

The Setup: Stand next to a wall, chair, desk, or other solid object to touch or grasp for balance. Stand with your feet hip-width apart, knees relaxed, and toes pointed forward. Shift your weight to your left leg, and lift your right foot off the ground. Keep both hips level rather than sinking into the left hip.

The Action: Slowly lift up onto the toes of your left foot by contracting your calf muscles. Keep your shoulders down and slightly back, your abdominals pulled in, and your head and neck in alignment with your spine. Look straight ahead, not down. Hold the top position for 2 seconds, then slowly lower your heel, taking a full 5 to 7 seconds for each repetition. Do all of your repetitions on your left leg before switching sides.

Stretching and De-Stressing

When you talk about exercising on the road, chances are you're referring to cardio workouts or strength training. But the third component of fitness — the most neglected one, stretching — is just as important, if not more important, for a traveler. Just because your heart isn't racing and you're not drenched in sweat doesn't mean you're not doing something vital for your body.

Part IV explains why stretching is so crucial when you're traveling and includes flexibility and relaxation exercises you can do just about anywhere. Chapter 13 covers basic stretches that will loosen you up, get your blood flowing, and leave you feeling rejuvenated. Chapter 14 features soothing, stress-reducing moves that blend yoga and tai chi.

13

Essential Stretches for the Fit Traveler

You've been squeezed into an airline seat, cramped behind the wheel of a car, stuffed in a tour bus for hours on end. By the time you set foot on solid ground, your muscles seem to have shrunk like blue jeans just out of the dryer. You've got that traveler's stiffness: the rigid walk, the tight neck, the tense shoulders, the achy lower back.

No one needs to stretch more than a weary traveler. Flexibility exercises can help you avoid much of the tightness and lethargy that come from sitting immobile in confined quarters. You can perform these exercises in your hotel room, at a highway rest stop, at the airport, even on the airplane. You'll feel invigorated and refreshed, and over the long haul you'll have better mobility, better posture, and a lower risk of back pain.

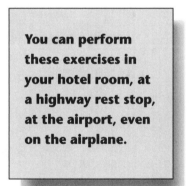

You can perform these exercises in your hotel room, at a highway rest stop, at the airport, even on the airplane.

The exercises in this chapter were selected by martial arts expert Tom Seabourne, who, at age 45, can still do the splits. Seabourne stretched in airports worldwide when he traveled as a member of the U.S. tae kwon do team. "I'd find a gate that didn't have a flight going out and hide behind the seats to stretch," Seabourne recalls. When he couldn't find an empty space, he'd perform his contortions in public. "People would stop and stare," says Seabourne, who would do the standing splits, with one leg propped straight up against the wall. "But I didn't care."

These days when he travels, Seabourne does a flexibility routine every night before he goes to bed. If there's not enough space on the floor, he'll stretch on the king-size bed. "When you do the splits on the bed, you sink down and you don't get as good a stretch," he says, "so I prop pillows under each of my ankles." Don't worry: This chapter doesn't include the splits or any other exercises requiring superhuman flexibility. The stretches are basic moves that just about anyone can manage, and you can do all of them standing up — no king-size bed required.

Preworkout Briefing

Here are some basic stretching guidelines.

- Stretch as often as you can, preferably at least once a day.

- Exhale as you slowly move into each position, hold the stretch for 10 to 15 seconds without bouncing, then relax.

- Stretch only to the point of mild tension, never teeth-clenching pain.

- If possible, stretch after your cardiovascular workout or at least after a cardio warm-up. Warmer muscles are more pliable than cold ones, so you'll be able to stretch farther.

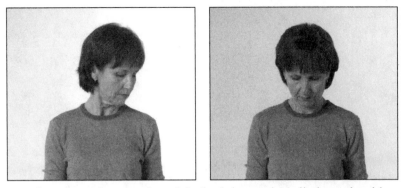

Stand or sit with your chest lifted, abdominals pulled in, shoulders relaxed, and both arms hanging down by your sides. Tilt your head to look down at your left hand, feeling a stretch in the right side of your neck. Hold, then look down at your right hand. Then return your neck to the center and drop your chin slowly toward your chest until you feel a stretch at the back of your neck. Move smoothly so you don't strain your neck.

SHOULDER STRETCH

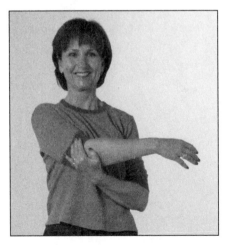

Sit or stand with your chest lifted, abdominals pulled in, and arms hanging down. Grab your right elbow with your left hand and gently pull it across your body. Stop when you feel tension in your shoulder. Hold, then switch sides.

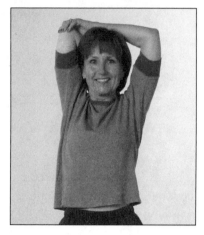 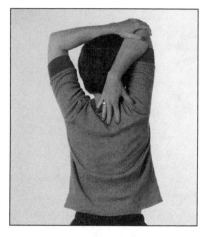

This move stretches both your shoulders and triceps.

Reach toward the ceiling with both hands, then bend your right elbow so that your right palm touches the back of your neck. Place your left hand on your right elbow and gently pull your right elbow back as your right hand slides slowly down your back. Stop when you feel tension in your shoulder and triceps. Hold, then switch sides.

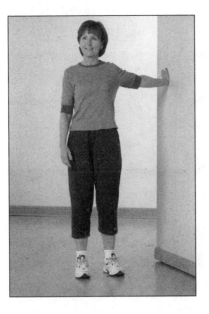

Chest stretches are key for long car trips. Holding the steering wheel with your shoulders slumped causes your chest muscles to tighten. Stretching these muscles will make you more comfortable by improving your posture and opening up your chest.

Stand with your left side next to a wall, and place your left hand on the wall at shoulder level with your elbow slightly bent. Slowly pivot your torso to the right until you feel a stretch on the left side of your chest. Hold, then switch sides.

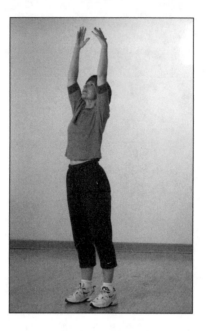

Your upper back muscles will become lax and lose tone if you sit still for long periods of time. Be like your house cat and stretch these muscles several times a day. You'll feel invigorated.

While sitting or standing, reach both arms as high as you can overhead so your fingers are almost touching at the peak of your reach. Look up, but not so far that you strain your neck. Feel the stretch in your upper back. Maintain a slight curve in your lower back throughout the stretch.

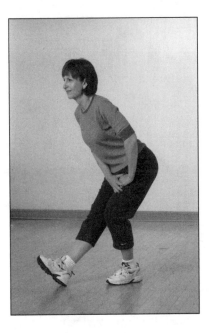

Tight hamstrings cause your pelvis to tilt backward, which can lead to stiff lower back muscles and, ultimately, lower back pain.

Stand with your feet slightly less than hip-width apart and bend slightly forward from your waist. Bend your left knee and place your palms, side by side, on your left thigh for support. Bring your right leg a few inches forward, heel on the floor and toes up. Drop your right hip back and lean your chest toward your right knee until you feel a gentle stretch in your right hamstring. Throughout the stretch, keep your back straight and abdominals pulled in. Hold, then switch legs.

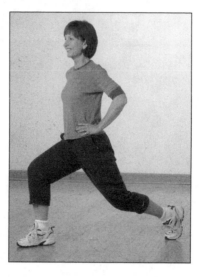

Your hip flexors are the muscles at the front of your thigh next to your groin. When you spend hours sitting, whether on an airplane or at a desk, these muscles shorten, causing your pelvis to tilt forward. The upshot: lower back pain. Lengthening your hip flexors will help you maintain perfect posture.

Stand with your feet together, knees slightly bent, and hands on your hips. Take a large step forward with your right foot, as if you are about to perform a lunge. Bend your right knee to almost 90 degrees, keeping your knee lined up over your big toe. Hold that position as you tilt your pelvis forward so you feel a stretch in your hip flexors. Hold, then switch legs.

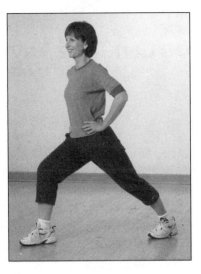

Calf stretches are particularly important if you do a lot of walking. These stretches help prevent injuries such as Achilles tendinitis (caused by tightening of the Achilles tendon) and plantar fascitis (caused by tightening of the tissue in the arch underneath the foot).

Stand with your feet together and both knees slightly bent. Take a big step forward with your right foot, as if you are about to perform a lunge. Bend your right knee to almost 90 degrees, with your knee lined up over your big toe. Keep your left heel on the floor as you lean into your lunge with your left leg almost straight. Feel the stretch in the back of your lower leg. Hold, then switch legs. Now switch legs again, but instead of holding your left leg straight, bend it until you feel a stretch.

14

Yoga You Can Take Anywhere

Delayed flights, overcrowded airports, lost luggage, maniac taxi drivers, misplaced hotel reservations — travel poses no shortage of stressful situations. Throw in high-pressure business meetings and after-hours schmoozing with clients, and by the end of the day, you're downright frazzled. You could always wind down with a martini in the lounge, but 15 minutes of yoga will probably do you even more good. Plus, you'll save the calories and the seven bucks.

The five exercises in this chapter are a blend of yoga and tai chi. You may find it most relaxing to perform the exercises in the quiet of your hotel room, although you can also do this routine at your hotel fitness center. Palm Springs trainer Scott Cole, who designed this workout, has even performed some of these moves on the airplane. "Other passengers ask what I'm doing, and usually I'll get someone else to do the moves with me," Cole says. "But then the flight attendant comes by with the cart and says, 'Excuse me, we're having meal service now.'"

> **You could always wind down with a martini in the lounge, but 15 minutes of yoga will probably do you even more good.**

Deep breathing — from your diaphragm, not your chest — is fundamental to feeling at ease during this workout. "The term 'getting centered' means just that: Put your energy back into your core or the center of your body," Cole says. "People naturally get red-faced, feel heart palpitations, and accumulate tension in their neck and shoulders when their energy has been out of center for too long." Relaxation is just a matter of letting your energy settle down. This workout will help you relax and rejuvenate for the next meeting, the next day, a good night's sleep, a night on the town, or the plane ride home.

Preworkout Briefing

Do these exercises in sequence or create your own workout with the moves you enjoy most. Perform each exercise two or three times if you like.

BENDING BEAR

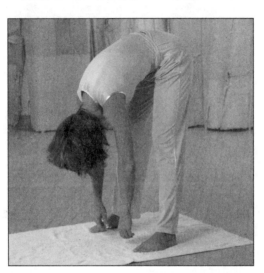

Adapted from an ancient tai chi–chi kung move, Bending Bear will relieve tension in your neck, back, shoulders, arms, hands, legs — essentially your entire body.

Stand with your feet hip-width apart or slightly wider, arms relaxed at your sides and knees slightly bent. Keeping your legs stabilized, bend at the waist and slowly let your torso fall all the way forward. Breathe naturally as you hang there with your back rounded, arms parallel to your legs, and fingertips nearing the floor. Feel your body relax with the natural force of gravity, and visualize energy flowing through all parts of your body. Breathe three to five full breaths without bouncing. Slowly roll up one vertebra at a time, counting backward from 5. With each stage — your lower back, middle back, upper back, and neck — you will feel an increasing sense of restoration.

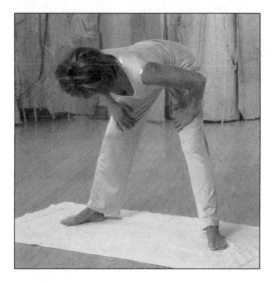

Martial arts like tai chi teach that locking your joints diminishes the flow of chi energy or life force. As you perform the Tabletop Stretch, keep your elbows and wrists relaxed and avoid lifting your shoulders.

Stand upright with your feet hip-width apart, inner thighs open, toes turned out to about 45 degrees. Place your hands on your quadriceps and your fingertips on your inner thighs, relaxing your elbows and shoulders. With your knees slightly bent and hands supported on your thighs, lean forward from your waist, using the natural force of gravity to ease into a flat-back position. Breathe deeply as you feel your legs relax and your spine lengthen.

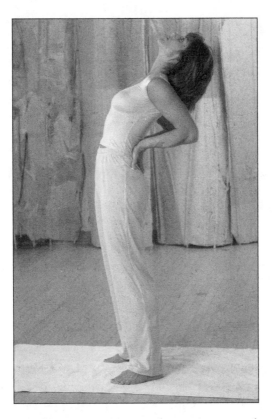

This yoga-inspired pose increases your lung capacity and is a great way to open up to new thoughts and attitudes. Plus, it just feels good.

Stand with your feet slightly apart for balance and breathe in slowly. As you inhale, place your hands into the small of your back, palms and fingertips down. As you exhale, gently begin to arch, lifting your breastbone and then easing back, supporting the arch with your arms and hands. Breathe easily as you continue to expand this posture, opening up through your hips, abs, and chest and relaxing your neck, face, and jaw. Enjoy the pose for 20 to 30 seconds. As you return to the start, focus on lifting from your breastbone. Your spine will follow and lengthen, so you will stand taller in the starting position.

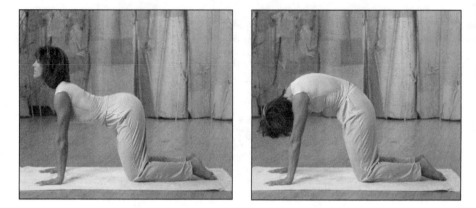

This version of the Yoga Cat Back combines the meditative flow of tai chi with the more stationary nature of traditional yoga. This move will improve your awareness, flexibility, and range of motion.

Move into an all-fours position, hands on the floor beneath your shoulders, elbows slightly bent, and knees on the floor directly below your hips. Working with gravity, let your back slowly arch. Inhale as you open your torso, looking up and out as your neck lengthens and your tailbone and butt ease out. Inhale fully, holding the position momentarily. As you exhale, round your back and neck forward, tucking your chin, tilting your pelvis forward, tucking your tailbone, and feeling a stretch throughout the back of your body. Don't linger in this position. Continue breathing, arching again on the inhale and returning to the tucked position on the exhale. Alternate between these positions for a minute or two.

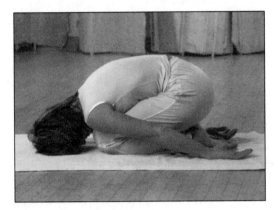

Often called the Baby or Infant Pose, the Child's Pose has beautiful symbolism. Feel free to place a pillow behind your knees or under your shins for comfort. With practice, however, you won't need these modifications.

From an all-fours position, ease your butt toward your heels, resting your arms at your sides with your fingertips back by your feet and your forehead on the floor. Open your knees a bit to facilitate easy breathing. If this pose is uncomfortable, shift your weight slightly forward, open your knees, and rest your forehead on your hands, elbows bent. Settle into the pose, feeling the tension release from your muscles and joints. The easier you breathe, the more your body will respond. Linger in this position as long as you want.

Final Thoughts

Travel always gives you perspective. Visit Houston in July and you'll have a greater understanding of the word *hot*. Visit Los Angeles any day of the year and you might groan less about traffic in your own city. Take a trip to Kyrgyzstan and you'll have new appreciation for one of North America's most magnificent innovations: quilted two-ply toilet paper.

Exercising during your travels only adds to your perspective, in ways that can bring new life to your fitness program once you return home.

After jogging in unfamiliar territory, never knowing quite where you are or whether you'll remember your way back, you might look more fondly on that same old route in your neighborhood; there's much to be said for the comforts of home. After grappling with creaky, outdated hotel gym machinery — or making do with a bed, a chair, and rubber tubing — you may return to your regular club with new enthusiasm for its shiny, well-oiled equipment. After you've managed to fit exercise into a frenzied, exhausting travel itinerary, you might realize that, at home, you have more time to work out than you'd thought.

Exercising in less-developed countries can offer a double dose of perspective. When David Negus returns from business trips to Africa and Southeast Asia, he's reminded how easy we have it in the developed world, where gyms are air-conditioned, weights labeled "30 pounds" actually weigh 30 pounds, and you're never too far from a protein smoothie. "I can't help but think of the gyms where the temperature is well over 90 and there's maybe one stand-up fan, the equipment is handmade, and the folks have only a basic rice-and-sauce meal to look forward to after their workout," says Negus, a deputy controller for a Washington, D.C.–based company. "But in these gyms you find people working out intensely, enjoying their time together, and maintaining physiques that are remarkable given the constraints they confront on a daily basis."

Sometimes your travels help you recognize how humdrum your workout routine has become. At home, it's easy to fall into a rut — to use the same weight machines in the same order, week after week, month after month, simply out of habit. But a trip may take the routine out of your routine. You may have no choice but to try new strength exercises or jog in the pool instead of swim laps. And you might find these new pursuits so enjoyable that you add them to your fitness repertoire at home.

Bike-racer Annelie Chapman resorted to climbing stairs in order to keep up her fitness while researching her doctoral dissertation in Moscow. But she found the workouts so effective that, after her return to Los Angeles, she started climbing stairs regularly in an eight-story building at a local university. "Having to improvise my training while traveling taught me to improvise at home, too," Chapman says. "Before, I'd get cranky when I couldn't ride my bike because it was too dark or rainy. Now, I'll just do something else. It's really liberating."

Of course, any new routine eventually becomes old hat. But if you're lucky, by the time that happens, you're ready to head off on your next trip.

Travel Workout Log

Index of Exercises

Useful Web Sites for the Fit Traveler

Travel Workout Log

Tracking your workouts on paper is a great way to keep yourself motivated on the road. (See Chapter 2 for details.) To get you started, here are some log pages adapted from *The Ultimate Workout Log* (Houghton Mifflin).

How to Use Your Log on the Road

Even if you record minimal information, it's a good idea to write *something* every day – and that includes days you don't exercise. This way, when you look back, you'll be able to distinguish between days you rested and days you were sick or injured. You'll have more clues as to how much training while traveling works best for you.

Goals for the Trip

Start each trip by identifying an exercise mission. Make your goals concrete, such as "swim 30 mins. every other day" or "climb hotel stairs after breakfast" or "lift weights twice a week." Set nutrition goals, too, such as "eat oatmeal for breakfast" or "order baked potato instead of fries."

Cardio Exercise

In this section you can record the time, distance, and intensity of your cardio workouts. Make a brief note about how hard you pushed, as a reminder to vary your intensity.

CARDIO EXERCISE	TIME/DISTANCE/INTENSITY	NOTES
swim	20 min. (25 laps)	took it easy
hotel steps	8 flights up, elevator down; 1 — 15 times	

Strength Training

In this section you can record your strength-training exercises, including how much weight you lifted, how many pushups you did, and the number of sets and repetitions you performed.

STRENGTH TRAINING	WT.	SETS	REPS	NUTRITION NOTES
military pushup		2	12	
lat pulldown	90	3	10	

Hours Slept

Note how long you slept so you can track whether you're getting enough rest.

Stretching

Check this box on the days you perform flexibility exercises.

Nutrition Notes

The purpose of this box isn't to record every calorie you ingest. Instead, focus on one or two nutrition goals at a time. For instance, note how many fruit and vegetable servings you ate in a day. Give yourself credit for choosing a turkey sub instead of a cheeseburger.

Wrap-up

Here's your chance to look back at the leg of the journey you just completed.

• **Goals:** It's easy to set goals, but it's even easier to forget you ever did. This section will keep you honest, forcing you to look back at the goals you set when you left.

• **Cardio, Strength, Nutrition Notes:** Assess your week as a whole and record any patterns. Record how many days you exercised in the Total Sessions boxes. Compare results to your weekly routine when at home.

Day 1

DATE _____

DAY OF WEEK _____

LOCATION _____

HOURS SLEPT ☐

STRETCHING ☐

CARDIO EXERCISE	TIME/DISTANCE/INTENSITY
_____	_____
_____	_____

NOTES

STRENGTH TRAINING	WT.	SETS	REPS
_____			
_____			
_____			
_____			
_____			
_____			
_____			
_____			
_____			

NUTRITION NOTES

Day 2

DATE _____

DAY OF WEEK _____

LOCATION _____

HOURS SLEPT ☐

STRETCHING ☐

CARDIO EXERCISE	TIME/DISTANCE/INTENSITY
_____	_____
_____	_____

NOTES

STRENGTH TRAINING	WT.	SETS	REPS
_____			
_____			
_____			
_____			
_____			
_____			
_____			
_____			
_____			

NUTRITION NOTES

Day 3

DATE _____

DAY OF WEEK _____

LOCATION _____

HOURS SLEPT ☐

STRETCHING ☐

CARDIO EXERCISE	TIME/DISTANCE/INTENSITY
_____	_____
_____	_____

NOTES

STRENGTH TRAINING	WT.	SETS	REPS
_____			
_____			
_____			
_____			
_____			
_____			
_____			
_____			
_____			

NUTRITION NOTES

Day 4

DATE _____

DAY OF WEEK _____

LOCATION _____

HOURS SLEPT ☐

STRETCHING ☐

CARDIO EXERCISE	TIME/DISTANCE/INTENSITY
_____	_____
_____	_____

NOTES

STRENGTH TRAINING	WT.	SETS	REPS
_____			
_____			
_____			
_____			
_____			
_____			
_____			
_____			
_____			

NUTRITION NOTES

Day 5

DATE _____

DAY OF WEEK _____

LOCATION _____

HOURS SLEPT [ ]

STRETCHING [ ]

CARDIO EXERCISE	TIME/DISTANCE/INTENSITY
_____	_____
_____	_____

NOTES

STRENGTH TRAINING	WT.	SETS	REPS
_____			
_____			
_____			
_____			
_____			
_____			
_____			
_____			
_____			

NUTRITION NOTES

Day 6

DATE _____

DAY OF WEEK _____

LOCATION _____

HOURS SLEPT [ ]

STRETCHING [ ]

CARDIO EXERCISE	TIME/DISTANCE/INTENSITY
_____	_____
_____	_____

NOTES

STRENGTH TRAINING	WT.	SETS	REPS
_____			
_____			
_____			
_____			
_____			
_____			
_____			
_____			
_____			

NUTRITION NOTES

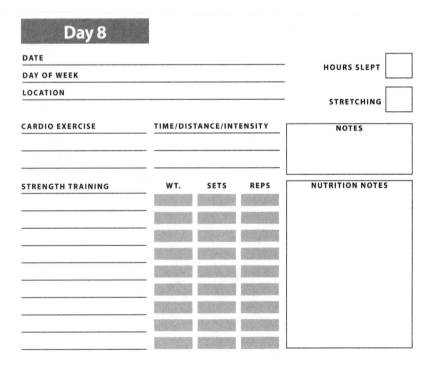

Day 7

DATE _____

DAY OF WEEK _____

LOCATION _____

HOURS SLEPT [   ]

STRETCHING [   ]

CARDIO EXERCISE	TIME/DISTANCE/INTENSITY
_____	_____
_____	_____

NOTES

STRENGTH TRAINING	WT.	SETS	REPS
_____			
_____			
_____			
_____			
_____			
_____			
_____			
_____			
_____			

NUTRITION NOTES

Day 8

DATE _____

DAY OF WEEK _____

LOCATION _____

HOURS SLEPT [   ]

STRETCHING [   ]

CARDIO EXERCISE	TIME/DISTANCE/INTENSITY
_____	_____
_____	_____

NOTES

STRENGTH TRAINING	WT.	SETS	REPS
_____			
_____			
_____			
_____			
_____			
_____			
_____			
_____			
_____			

NUTRITION NOTES

Day 9

DATE _____

DAY OF WEEK _____

LOCATION _____

HOURS SLEPT [ ]

STRETCHING [ ]

CARDIO EXERCISE	TIME/DISTANCE/INTENSITY
_____	_____
_____	_____

NOTES

STRENGTH TRAINING	WT.	SETS	REPS
_____			
_____			
_____			
_____			
_____			
_____			
_____			
_____			
_____			

NUTRITION NOTES

Day 10

DATE _____

DAY OF WEEK _____

LOCATION _____

HOURS SLEPT [ ]

STRETCHING [ ]

CARDIO EXERCISE	TIME/DISTANCE/INTENSITY
_____	_____
_____	_____

NOTES

STRENGTH TRAINING	WT.	SETS	REPS
_____			
_____			
_____			
_____			
_____			
_____			
_____			
_____			
_____			

NUTRITION NOTES

Day 11

DATE _____

DAY OF WEEK _____

LOCATION _____

HOURS SLEPT [ ]

STRETCHING [ ]

CARDIO EXERCISE	TIME/DISTANCE/INTENSITY
_____	_____
_____	_____

NOTES

STRENGTH TRAINING	WT.	SETS	REPS
_____			
_____			
_____			
_____			
_____			
_____			
_____			
_____			
_____			

NUTRITION NOTES

Day 12

DATE _____

DAY OF WEEK _____

LOCATION _____

HOURS SLEPT [ ]

STRETCHING [ ]

CARDIO EXERCISE	TIME/DISTANCE/INTENSITY
_____	_____
_____	_____

NOTES

STRENGTH TRAINING	WT.	SETS	REPS
_____			
_____			
_____			
_____			
_____			
_____			
_____			
_____			
_____			

NUTRITION NOTES

Day 13

DATE _____

DAY OF WEEK _____

LOCATION _____

HOURS SLEPT ☐

STRETCHING ☐

CARDIO EXERCISE	TIME/DISTANCE/INTENSITY
_____	_____
_____	_____

NOTES

STRENGTH TRAINING	WT.	SETS	REPS
_____			
_____			
_____			
_____			
_____			
_____			
_____			
_____			
_____			

NUTRITION NOTES

Day 14

DATE _____

DAY OF WEEK _____

LOCATION _____

HOURS SLEPT ☐

STRETCHING ☐

CARDIO EXERCISE	TIME/DISTANCE/INTENSITY
_____	_____
_____	_____

NOTES

STRENGTH TRAINING	WT.	SETS	REPS
_____			
_____			
_____			
_____			
_____			
_____			
_____			
_____			
_____			

NUTRITION NOTES

Day 15

DATE _____

DAY OF WEEK _____

LOCATION _____

HOURS SLEPT ☐

STRETCHING ☐

CARDIO EXERCISE	TIME/DISTANCE/INTENSITY
_____	_____
_____	_____

NOTES

STRENGTH TRAINING	WT.	SETS	REPS
_____			
_____			
_____			
_____			
_____			
_____			
_____			
_____			
_____			

NUTRITION NOTES

Day 16

DATE _____

DAY OF WEEK _____

LOCATION _____

HOURS SLEPT ☐

STRETCHING ☐

CARDIO EXERCISE	TIME/DISTANCE/INTENSITY
_____	_____
_____	_____

NOTES

STRENGTH TRAINING	WT.	SETS	REPS
_____			
_____			
_____			
_____			
_____			
_____			
_____			
_____			
_____			

NUTRITION NOTES

Index of Exercises

The following list organizes exercises according to the main muscle groups strengthened.

Useful Web Sites for the Fit Traveler

Where to buy fitness products you can pack

Amazon.com   The online megabookstore offers a variety of workout logs with reviews to help you choose.

Bodytrends.com   This site sells heart-rate monitors, pedometers, exercise tubing, jump ropes, CD-player belts, and other handy fitness products.

Bodytronics.com   This is another place to shop for motivational tools such as pedometers, heart-rate monitors, and sports watches.

Camelbak.com   The company that made the water bottle obsolete for outdoor exercise offers hydration packs (water pouches you wear on your back) for walking, hiking, biking, skiing, and other activities.

Collagevideo.com   The country's largest workout video catalog also sells CDs designed for walking, jogging, and stationary biking, along with accessories such as workout logs and exercise tubing.

Dynamixmusic.com   Here you can find CDs designed to keep you motivated — or relaxed — during yoga, jogging, walking, aquatic exercise, and other workouts.

Hydrofit.com   This site features accessories for aquatic workouts, including webbed gloves, athletic shoes designed for water, and videotapes and instruction manuals that demonstrate aerobic and muscle-conditioning moves for the pool.

Hydrotone.com   In addition to offering illustrated instructions for cardio moves, this site sells products to make aquatic workouts more challenging, such as dumbbells and gloves.

Performbetter.com   This online catalog specializes in strength-training and rehab devices, including tubing, pushup equipment, stretching devices, books, and videos.

Spriproducts.com   The Spri catalog sells exercise tubing and bands in all shapes and sizes, as well as travel workout videos, exercise mats, and other fitness products.

Zura.com   This is the place to buy inflatable kickboards and pull buoys for your swim workouts on the road.

Where to find health clubs, jogging routes, and pools on the road

Ballyfitness.com   Use this site to locate Bally Total Fitness clubs in the United States and Canada.

24hourfitness.com   The "club finder" feature lets you locate some 400 24-Hour Fitness clubs worldwide and explains the company's guest policies.

Goldsgym.com   Search by Zip Code to find the Gold's Gym location nearest you and get an instant map online.

Healthclubs.com   This site features about 6,000 clubs in the United States and abroad, complete with maps and driving directions.

Kilmartin.com   Laugh out loud as you read comedian and swimmer Laurie Kilmartin's reviews of swimming pools nationwide.

Nutricise.com   The "Gym Locator" in this fitness and nutrition site includes 10,000 health clubs nationwide. The site also features an in-depth report on airline meals.

Runnersworld.com   The online version of *Runner's World* magazine leads you to running trails, clubs, and stores in more than 80 cities worldwide.

Swimmersguide.com   A remarkable resource, this site gives detailed information on more than 9,000 full-size pools in more than 90 countries.

Ymca.net   Use this site to locate thousands of YMCA locations in the United States and around the world.

Where to find useful fitness and nutrition information

Acefitness.org   The nonprofit American Council on Exercise, the world's largest organization of fitness professionals, offers online information about strength training, cardiovascular workouts, stretching, and other forms of exercise. ACE's monthly newsletter, "ACE Fitness Matters," helps separate fitness fact from fiction.

Cspinet.org   The nonprofit Center for Science in the Public Interest is a wealth of valuable, sometimes shocking, nutritional information about the food we eat. CSPI's "Eating Smart Restaurant Guide" is essential for travelers, and its "Nutrition Action Healthletter" will boost your nutritional knowledge.

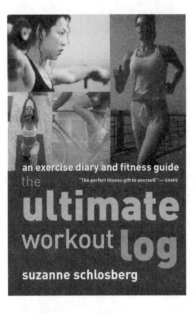